The Self Heal Bible

The Complete Guide to Barbara O'Neill's Teachings | Natural Remedies and Herbal Recipes to Restore Your Body's Self-Healing Power

Mia Williams

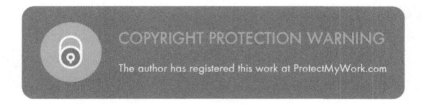

Table of Contents

FOREWORD

Hey there! So, you're probably holding this book, thinking, "Who's Mia Williams and why should I listen to her?" I've got a story to tell you – mine. It's not about wild adventures, but a journey of quiet, deep change that touches the heart and shows just how smart our bodies can be when it comes to healing.

Picture this: my life was kind of stuck in a rut, feeling like real health was some fairy tale. I was wandering through a maze of standard health tips that didn't help at all. Then, everything started to shift, not with some big bang, but with an eye-opening moment at Misty Mountain Lifestyle Retreat. This place, where the earth's gentle whispers meet Barbara O'Neill's sage advice, was where everything clicked. Barbara's insights, so deep yet so soothing, started to change me from the inside out. Surrounded by nature's peace, I realized that being healthy isn't just about not being sick – it's about living a life brimming with vitality, something we're all meant to do.

Every day at Misty Mountain peeled away my doubts and discomfort, showing me a newer, more vibrant me – full of energy, thinking clearly, and feeling a deep bond with the natural world. This wasn't a solo trip; I was part of a whole crowd of us looking for a glimmer of hope on our health journey. Driven by the big shifts in my own life and all that Barbara shared, I dove headfirst into natural healing. My trips to Misty Mountain turned into my own kind of sacred journey, a time to grow and really soak in this whole wellness vibe that had given me so much.

And now, here I am, sharing this book with you, buzzing with excitement and fired up about all the ways we can transform. With a nod to Barbara O'Neill's treasure trove of wisdom, I'm inviting you to dig in, dream big, and wrap your arms around the magic of natural healing. So, who am I? Just someone who's been down the road you're about to take. I've been through the lows of feeling sick and the highs of finding my spark again. I'm not just passing along some tips; I'm sharing a story of how nature and our own grit can truly turn things around. With a big welcome and a heart full of stories, I'm here to take this trip with you. Let's journey through the world of health and wellness, led by Barbara O'Neill's timeless wisdom and the life-changing experiences at Misty Mountain Lifestyle Retreats. Here's to a fresh start, a new chapter where every page is a step toward feeling great. Ready to dive in? Let's do this with all the excitement, curiosity, and the thrill of discovering what's possible.

Take care,

Mia Williams

INTRODUCTION

A huge thanks for letting this book be a part of your journey. What you're holding isn't just a bunch of pages—it's a door to a whole new you. This isn't just about tips and tricks; it's a blend of knowledge and wisdom that's all about helping you find a deeper, more in-sync kind of health and happiness. This book is like a handshake between your own wish to feel amazing and some of the best, time-honored healing vibes out there. By starting this journey, you're already showing you're not just about getting by—you want to shine. Every bit of this book is packed with chances to turn your view of health inside out, nudging you to see just how incredible your body is at bouncing back and blooming when you treat it right.

So, what's going to click with you? Which bits of wisdom will you weave into your day-to-day? How will the stories and strategies here open your eyes to new ways of looking after yourself? That's the beauty of it—it's all up to you. Everyone who reads this book will connect with different parts, but what we all share is this quest to live life full throttle.

This book is also a big high five to the idea of choosing—choosing to learn, to change, to dive into this health journey with all your heart. As you flip through these pages, think of it as a conversation. Be curious, ask questions, and figure out how what you're reading fits with your life and dreams. You picking up this book shows you're ready to get real about feeling great. Think of it as your buddy and mentor, packed with insights that can shake things up, offer comfort, and maybe even confirm what you've always known deep down. It's here to walk with you as you discover not just the ins and outs of holistic health, but also a lot about yourself. So, come on—let's take this leap. Get ready for all the learning, growth, and ah-ha moments ahead. This book is more than just words; it's the first step on a path that could totally remix your approach to life, love, and wellness. Welcome to the beginning of something awesome—a tale of health, healing, and how tough we all are. Let's kick this off, together.

Overview of Barbara O'Neill's Philosophy

Barbara O'Neill is all about celebrating the body's own superhero powers to fix itself, with a little help from Mother Nature. She's convinced that being healthy is what our bodies do best, and from this point of view, she dives into everything from what we eat to how we deal with stress and emotions. Imagine your body as this incredible lab, all set to heal and thrive—but it needs the right stuff to work with. Clean air, enough sleep, and the right kind of food are key. Barbara points out how we've turned the smallest health hiccups into big deals that need medication, when really, our bodies could handle a lot of this on their own if we just got back to basics.

Tired of ads pushing the latest pill? Barbara's with you. She questions our obsession with quick fixes and champions getting back in touch with what our bodies really need. Nutrition is her big thing. She's all about foods that are just right for us—think fruits, veggies, grains, nuts, and seeds that pack a punch with vitamins, minerals, and those all-important plant goodies. She's backed by studies showing how these foods can be our allies against things like cancer and heart disease. Processed foods and too much meat? Not so much. According to Barbara, they're the villains behind a lot of health issues, which makes wholesome food the real deal for healing and staying well.

Detoxing is another part of her plan. It's about clearing out the nasties from our environment, what we eat, and our lifestyle choices that bog down our body's healing vibes. Stuff like fasting, juicing, and hitting the sauna can help kick toxins to the curb, letting our bodies get back to their best. But Barbara doesn't stop at just the physical stuff. She knows that real health is about the whole package—body, mind, and spirit. She's all about feeding every part of ourselves with good food, exercise, enough rest, and stress-busting activities that make us feel whole and happy, like meditation, deep breaths, and spending time in nature.

Learning to look after all parts of ourselves is her big-picture way to a healthier life. And here's the best part: Barbara wants to power us up with knowledge. It's not just about doing what you're told; it's understanding why and how making certain choices can totally turn your health around. She's like the ultimate coach, cheering us on to take control of our health journey and drive ourselves toward something incredible.

The Importance of Holistic Health

Diving into holistic health with Barbara O'Neill is like finding a hidden map to treasure island, but instead of gold, the chest is filled with secrets to feeling amazing. She invites us to see health as this big, beautiful picture where everything—how we move, think, and feel—is connected, creating a kind of harmony that makes us glow from the inside out. Barbara doesn't just skim the surface; she goes deep, showing us that true health is this awesome mix of energy, vitality, and balance.

Imagine you're a puzzle, right? Each piece represents something different about you—your habits, your thoughts, your emotions. If one piece is missing, like maybe you're all about the gym but you don't give a hoot about how stressed you are, the puzzle isn't complete. It's like trying to see the whole picture with a chunk gone. Barbara opens our eyes to this, teaching us to aim for a balance, a perfect fit where every aspect of our well-being clicks together.

She talks about how taking care of our bodies is more than just hitting the gym; it's about what we eat, how we sleep, and even how we breathe. She stresses eating right and getting enough z's as the basics of feeling good. And it's not just about the body. If your mind's a mess with stress or negativity, it's going to mess with your health, too. Barbara's all about clearing the mental clutter with things like mindfulness and keeping good vibes in our relationships, kind of like keeping a garden weeded so the good stuff can grow. The cool thing about looking at health this way is how everything affects everything else. Eat better, and you might just find you're happier. Get a handle on stress, and watch your physical health get a boost. It's like a domino effect of awesomeness. Barbara nudges us to make smart, daily choices—choosing real food, finding moments for quiet, getting enough sleep, and building strong bonds with others. These steps aren't just good for us on their own; they work together, making our lives richer and more vibrant.

Barbara's not saying we have to be perfect. It's about taking steps, big or small, towards a more balanced, joyful life. Ready to put your puzzle together and see the amazing picture it makes? Barbara's guiding us, one caring step at a time, towards a life filled with energy and peace. Let's take this journey with open minds and hearts, connecting more deeply with ourselves and the world around us.

How This Guide Meets the Readers' Needs

This guide is crafted with a keen eye on what you, the reader, truly need: *specificity, practicality, and reliability.* We've all been there, wading through heaps of information, seeking those golden nuggets that can genuinely make a difference in our lives. This guide aims to be that treasure trove for you, distilling Barbara O'Neill's profound teachings into something you can actually use, something that resonates with your daily life. Let's break down how this guide is tailored to meet those needs, ensuring it's not just another read, but a practical companion on your journey to holistic health.

Specificity: *Ever felt lost in the vague "just eat healthy" advice?* This guide cuts through the ambiguity, diving into the "what," "why," and "how" of natural healing. It's about providing clear, detailed insights into specific remedies, dietary suggestions, and lifestyle adjustments—all inspired by Barbara O'Neill's rich experience. *Want to know the exact steps to prepare a detoxifying juice, or the types of exercises that harmonize with natural healing principles?* We've got you covered. This guide is your roadmap, marked with clear signposts, guiding you through the maze of natural health towards actionable paths.

Practicality: What good is information if you can't use it? The essence of this guide's practicality lies in its integration into your daily routines. We understand the modern-day challenges of balancing work, family, and personal time, which is why this guide is designed to fit into your life, not the other way around. From quick, nutritious recipes that fit into your busy morning to stress-relief techniques for your office break, we provide strategies that blend seamlessly into your day. It's about making holistic health attainable and manageable, ensuring that the steps you take are not just effective but also enjoyable.

Reliability: In a world brimming with health advice, discerning what to trust can be overwhelming. This guide stands as a beacon of reliability, rooted in Barbara O'Neill's evidence-based teachings and enriched with the latest research in natural health. Each recommendation, each piece of advice, is backed by a commitment to accuracy and depth. It's information you can trust, giving you the confidence to make informed decisions about your health. Whether you're exploring a remedy for the first time or seeking to deepen your understanding of a holistic practice, this guide offers a solid foundation, ensuring that the steps you take towards better health are grounded in knowledge and wisdom. I would like to point out, however, that although every research has been done on the accuracy of the topics, there is no one-size-fits-all in caring for one's health. Therefore, it is strongly discouraged to use the advice given in this guide without the supervision of a trusted health care professional.

In essence, this guide is more than just a collection of health tips—it's a dynamic, living resource tailored to your needs. It's about providing *specific, practical, and reliable* guidance that empowers you to embrace holistic health in a way that's meaningful and sustainable. Barbara O'Neill's teachings come alive in these pages, offering you a hand to hold as you navigate the journey to a healthier, more vibrant you. *So, are you ready to dive in and transform these teachings into actions?* Let's embark on this journey together, embracing a healthier, more vibrant version of yourself.

Book 1: The Fundamentals of Natural Healing

Understanding Natural Healing

Welcome to the world of natural healing—a journey back to the basics, where the power of nature and the wisdom of ages converge to offer a path to health and wellness. It's a realm where the body's innate healing capabilities are honored and nurtured, tapping into the natural resources that surround us to foster recovery and well-being. *But what exactly is natural healing, and what principles guide this ancient yet timeless approach to health?* Let's dive in.

Principles of Natural Healing

Natural healing, at its core, is an approach to health and wellness that utilizes the body's inherent ability to heal itself. It eschews synthetic drugs and invasive procedures in favor of natural remedies, lifestyle adjustments, and holistic practices. This method encompasses a wide array of practices, including herbal medicine, nutrition, physical movement, and mind-body therapies, all aimed at restoring balance and harmony within the body. It's a holistic philosophy that views the individual as a complete entity, interconnecting the physical, emotional, mental, and sometimes spiritual aspects of well-being. The principles of natural healing are grounded in the belief that the body, when provided with the right conditions, can heal itself from within. Here are some foundational tenets:

- **The Holistic Approach:** Natural healing recognizes the individual as an integrated whole. Health is not merely the absence of disease but a state of complete physical, mental, and emotional well-being. This principle emphasizes the interconnectedness of the body, mind, and spirit, advocating for treatments that address all aspects of the individual.

- **Prevention is Key:** It places a strong emphasis on disease prevention through maintaining a healthy lifestyle, diet, and environment. The idea is to prevent illness from taking root, rather than fighting diseases after they occur.

- **The Healing Power of Nature:** This principle is based on the belief that nature has the power to heal. Natural healing promotes the use of natural remedies—such as herbs, foods, and water—and practices like sunlight exposure and grounding, which are thought to restore health.

- **First Do No Harm:** Natural healing practices strive to be non-invasive and have minimal side effects. The aim is to support the body's healing processes without causing further harm, using the gentlest interventions necessary to stimulate recovery.

- **Identify and Treat the Cause:** Rather than just alleviating symptoms, natural healing seeks to identify and address the underlying causes of illness. It looks beyond the symptoms to the root of the problem, aiming for a more permanent solution to health issues.

- **Education and Empowerment:** An essential aspect of natural healing is educating individuals about their health and how their choices impact their well-being. It empowers people to take an active role in their health journey, fostering a sense of responsibility for their own well-being.

- **Healing is a Personal Journey:** Recognizing that each person is unique, natural healing emphasizes personalized care. Treatments and practices are tailored to meet the individual's specific needs, preferences, and conditions, acknowledging that what works for one person may not work for another.

By embracing these principles, natural healing offers a path to wellness that is aligned with the rhythms of the natural world and the unique needs of the individual. It's a journey back to the roots of wellness, inviting us to reconnect with the healing powers that lie both within us and in the natural environment around us. As we delve deeper into the realms of natural remedies, nutrition, and holistic practices, we'll explore how these principles come to life, guiding us toward a state of balanced, vibrant health.

History and Evolution of Naturopathy

The journey of natural healing is as ancient as humanity itself, with its modern incarnation, naturopathy, weaving through history like a green thread, connecting the wisdom of the past with the knowledge of the present. Naturopathy, or naturopathic medicine, emerges from the holistic principles of natural healing, embracing the body's power to heal itself through the support of nature's remedies and the balance of mind, body, and spirit. Its history and evolution are a fascinating tale of tradition, science, and the enduring quest for holistic wellness.

Naturopathy's roots can be traced back to the healing practices of ancient civilizations, including the Greeks, Egyptians, and Indians, who all recognized the medicinal properties of plants, the importance of diet, and the holistic nature of health.

Hippocrates, a figure often dubbed the *"Father of Medicine,"* espoused many principles that would later be fundamental to naturopathy, including the concept that disease results from natural causes and the healing power of nature. The term "naturopathy" was coined in the late 19th century, a period marked by a burgeoning interest in natural health and healing practices. It was during this time that the Industrial Revolution's advances brought about significant changes in lifestyle and diet, leading to a rise in chronic illnesses. In response, a counter-movement emerged, championing the return to natural living and healing methods. One of the pivotal figures in naturopathy's early development was Benedict Lust, who is often referred to as the *"Father of U.S. Naturopathy."* After experiencing healing through natural means in Germany, Lust brought these ideas to the United States, where he founded the first school of naturopathy in 1902. His work helped establish naturopathy as a distinct profession, emphasizing the body's innate healing ability and the importance of preventive care.

Throughout the 20th century, naturopathy faced challenges and opposition from the burgeoning pharmaceutical industry and the mainstream medical establishment. However, it continued to evolve and grow, incorporating scientific research into traditional practices and expanding its therapeutic toolkit to include a wide range of natural therapies such as herbal medicine, homeopathy, physical therapies, and nutrition. The latter half of the century saw a resurgence of interest in naturopathy and holistic health, fueled by growing disillusionment with conventional medicine's focus on symptom management and invasive treatments. This renewed interest led to the establishment of accredited naturopathic colleges, professional standards, and licensing in several countries, bringing naturopathy into the realm of recognized and regulated health professions.

Today, naturopathy stands at the intersection of ancient wisdom and modern science, offering a comprehensive approach to health and healing that is both preventive and curative. It emphasizes the importance of understanding the individual as a whole, tailoring treatments to the person, not just the disease. Naturopathic practitioners work in various settings, from private clinics to integrated healthcare systems, collaborating with other health professionals to provide holistic care. The evolution of naturopathy reflects humanity's enduring quest for balance and wellness, a testament to the belief in the healing power of nature and the body's potential for self-repair. As we continue to face health challenges in the modern world, the principles of naturopathy offer a guiding light, reminding us of the importance of harmony between nature, body, and spirit in the pursuit of lasting health.

Within the tapestry of naturopathy's evolution, Barbara O'Neill emerges as a beacon of knowledge and inspiration, significantly enriching the modern landscape of natural healing. Through her seminars, writings, and hands-on health retreats, she has played a pivotal role in educating both the public and health professionals about the fundamentals of natural healing and the importance of dietary and lifestyle interventions. Her emphasis on the body's innate ability to heal itself, given the right support through nutrition, herbal medicine, detoxification, and stress management, echoes the core principles of naturopathy and has helped bring this healing modality to a wider audience. *Curious to know more about its outstanding contribution in the world of natural healing?* Then you'll love diving into the next section focusing on this.

Barbara O'Neill's Contributions

Barbara O'Neill's journey into the realm of natural healing is a testament to the transformative power of nature and the profound resilience of the human body. Her story begins with a personal challenge—a severe health issue faced by her first child, which conventional medicine struggled to address. This pivotal moment ignited Barbara's quest for alternative solutions and marked the beginning of her deep dive into the world of natural healing. As a trained nurse with a profound love for nature, Barbara was uniquely positioned to bridge the gap between conventional health wisdom and the often-overlooked virtues of natural remedies. Her approach was both scientific and experimental, driven by a relentless pursuit of knowledge and a mother's determination to find healing for her child. Turning to the vast expanse of natural healing literature, Barbara absorbed every piece of information she could find, applying her learnings with careful consideration and witnessing firsthand the efficacy of natural treatments.

Her experiments, conducted with the loving intention of a mother and the precision of a nurse, brought to light a fundamental truth that would define her life's work: natural treatments, when applied correctly, are not only effective but also come with the added benefit of being free from the dangerous side effects often associated with conventional medications. Barbara's deep-seated belief in the Creator and the intricate design of creation led her to a profound realization—the body is inherently equipped with the capacity to heal itself, given the right conditions. This revelation transformed her role from a caregiver to an educator, dedicating her life to teaching others how to create the conditions conducive to self-healing. Her philosophy underscores a critical distinction: she is not the healer; the true healer is the body itself. Barbara's mission is to illuminate the path to wellness, empowering individuals with the knowledge and tools necessary to support their body's natural healing processes.

Her teachings are anchored in the principle that health and healing are accessible to everyone, provided they understand and apply the natural laws that govern the body's operation. Barbara O'Neill's contributions to natural healing go beyond her success stories; they encapsulate a message of hope, empowerment, and a return to the basics of health care. Through her seminars, publications, and retreats, she has become a beacon for those seeking to reclaim their health naturally, advocating for a holistic approach that harmonizes the physical, mental, and spiritual aspects of well-being. In essence, Barbara O'Neill's legacy in the field of natural healing is not just about the remedies she advocates for but the empowerment she offers to individuals worldwide. She teaches that by understanding the conditions necessary for health, anyone can tap into the innate healing capabilities of their own body, fostering a life of wellness and harmony with nature's design.

Understanding the Body's Mastery of Self-Healing

In 1690, Robert Boyle, a pioneer of the scientific method, marveled at the *"exquisite structure"* of the human body, a sentiment that rings just as true today. This divine architecture, much like a meticulously designed mansion we are privileged to inhabit, encapsulates not just the brilliance of its construction but also its innate capacity for self-repair and renewal. This chapter ventures into the heart of the body's natural healing abilities, unveiling the philosophical depth and practical implications of this remarkable feature of our existence. The question that presents itself with pressing urgency is this: *If our bodies are indeed equipped with such profound self-healing capabilities, why does sickness persist so prevalently among us?* The answer lies not in the body's inadequacies but in our own. The body, when accorded the right conditions, unfailingly embarks on the path to healing itself. However, a glaring paradox emerges in our modern existence—we, who have mastered the complexities of the most intricate machines and technologies, find ourselves at a loss when it comes to understanding the basic operations of our own biological machinery.

At the core of our exploration is the Carbon Cycle, a testament to the eternal dance of life, death, and rebirth that governs existence. This cycle, fundamental to the natural world, mirrors the processes within our bodies, where growth and decay coexist in a delicate balance, sustained by the diligent work of microorganisms. These tiny architects of life play an indispensable role in recycling dead matter into nutrients that fuel the continuation of life—a process as critical within the confines of our bodies as it is in the vast expanses of nature. Our journey delves deep into the realm of these microorganisms, especially those residing in the gastrointestinal tract, a bustling metropolis where nutrients are assimilated, and health is profoundly influenced. Here, in this intricate ecosystem, microorganisms labor tirelessly, breaking down food, synthesizing essential vitamins, and fortifying our defenses against disease. Their work underscores the symbiotic relationship we share with the microbial world, a partnership foundational to our health and survival. Yet, in the whirlwind of modern life, we find ourselves increasingly alienated from the natural cycles that sustain us. Our lifestyles, often disconnected from the rhythms of the natural world, neglect the basic needs of our bodies, leading us into a maze of preventable illnesses. This disconnection, coupled with a pervasive ignorance about the body's inherent needs and healing processes, has precipitated a health crisis of epidemic proportions. *"Sickness as No Accident"* posits that the key to unlocking our healing potential lies in reestablishing our connection with the natural world and gaining a profound understanding of the body's natural needs. By aligning our lifestyles with the principles that govern life and health—embracing the nourishment, rest, and care our bodies require—we can initiate a profound transformation in our health landscape.

The Microbial Metropolis Within Us

The revelation that our bodies harbor a vast community of microorganisms, outnumbering human cells, has dramatically shifted our understanding of what it means to be human. This diverse ecosystem, known as the human microbiome, comprises bacteria, viruses, fungi, and other microscopic entities that reside on our skin, in our mouths, and most prolifically, within our guts. Far from being mere passengers, these microorganisms play crucial roles in our health and development, challenging the traditional view of the human body as an isolated organism. Instead, we are now seen as complex ecosystems where human and microbial cells coexist in a delicate balance, influencing everything from digestion and immune function to mental health and disease susceptibility. This chapter delves into the intricacies of the human microbiome, shedding light on its composition, functions, and impact on our well-being, thereby underscoring the paradigm shift in understanding our bodies and the microscopic life forms that inhabit them.

Unveiling the Human Microbiome

The human microbiome refers to the collective genome of all microorganisms living in and on the human body. The terms "microflora" and "microbiota" are often used interchangeably, yet they bear distinct meanings. Microflora traditionally refers to the microscopic plants living within a region, an outdated term when applied to the human body. Microbiota, on the other hand, accurately describes the community of bacteria, viruses, fungi, and protozoa that inhabit our bodies.

Microorganisms in the human body are not uniformly distributed; rather, they colonize specific niches, from the dry and nutrient-poor environment of the skin to the nutrient-rich and densely populated gastrointestinal tract. The gut microbiota is the most studied, known for its complex interaction with the host, influencing health and disease. It's estimated that the human gut alone is home to over 100 trillion microorganisms, outnumbering human cells by a factor of ten to one. This diversity is not just in numbers but in the variety of species, with several thousand species cohabiting in the human body, each playing unique roles in health and disease.

The ubiquity and diversity of microorganisms within us highlight the significance of the microbiome in human physiology. From aiding digestion to synthesizing vitamins and regulating the immune system, the microbiome's functions are critical to our survival and well-being. Understanding this complex microbial ecosystem not only provides insights into human health but also unveils new avenues for treating diseases. Continuing from the established foundation, we now delve into the specifics of the gastrointestinal tract's microbial community, its protective functions, and its vital role in nutrient absorption and health maintenance, addressing dysbiosis and strategies for fostering a healthy microbiome.

The Gastrointestinal Tract: A Hub of Microbial Activity

The gastrointestinal (GI) tract stands as the epicenter of microbial activity within the human body, hosting a complex community of microorganisms that play pivotal roles in digestion, nutrient synthesis, and the immune system's development. Microorganisms within the GI tract are indispensable for breaking down complex carbohydrates, fibers, and other indigestible compounds, facilitating nutrient absorption and energy extraction from food. Additionally, gut microbiota synthesize essential vitamins, such as vitamin B and K, which are crucial for blood coagulation, bone health, and energy metabolism. The gut microbiota is instrumental in shaping the immune system. By distinguishing between commensal (beneficial) and pathogenic (harmful) microbes, it educates the immune system to react appropriately to different stimuli. This interaction helps in developing a balanced immune response, essential for preventing autoimmunity and fighting off infections.

Guardians of the Gut

Gut microorganisms serve as guardians against harmful pathogens through various mechanisms, including competitive exclusion, strengthening of the gut barrier, and modulation of the immune system. By occupying niches and utilizing available nutrients, beneficial microbes prevent the colonization of pathogens, a phenomenon known as competitive exclusion. Furthermore, they reinforce the gut barrier, preventing harmful substances and bacteria from entering the bloodstream. Gut microbiota also play a crucial role in modulating the immune system, enhancing its ability to identify and combat pathogens. This involves the production of substances that stimulate immune responses and the regulation of inflammation, crucial for maintaining gut health and preventing systemic diseases. The symbiotic relationship between humans and their gut microbiota extends to nutrient absorption. This section examines how gut microbes contribute to the breakdown of complex molecules and the absorption of nutrients, influencing the host's nutritional status and energy yield from food. Gut microbiota possess enzymes that humans lack, enabling the breakdown of complex carbohydrates, proteins, and lipids. This process not only aids in nutrient absorption but also produces short-chain fatty acids (SCFAs), beneficial compounds that serve as energy sources for the host and protect against diseases like colorectal cancer. The efficiency of nutrient absorption and energy yield from food is significantly influenced by the composition of the gut microbiota. A diverse and balanced microbiome enhances the host's ability to extract nutrients from the diet, impacting overall health and well-being.

Dysbiosis and Disease

Dysbiosis, an imbalance in the gut microbiota, is associated with a range of diseases, including inflammatory bowel disease, obesity, diabetes, and certain cancers. Factors such as antibiotics, diet, stress, and environmental influences can disrupt the delicate balance of the gut microbiota, leading to dysbiosis. This imbalance can compromise the gut barrier, enhance inflammation, and predispose individuals to various diseases. Dysbiosis has been linked to several chronic conditions, highlighting the importance of a balanced microbiome for disease prevention and health maintenance.

Therefore, maintaining a healthy gut microbiota is crucial for overall health. Incorporating prebiotics and probiotics through diet and avoiding unnecessary antibiotics can significantly influence the composition and health of the gut microbiota. Lifestyle changes, such as regular exercise and stress reduction, also play a vital role. Emerging research on fecal microbiota transplantation (FMT) shows promise in treating conditions like Clostridium difficile infection, indicating the potential of microbiome manipulation in disease treatment.

The exploration of the human microbiome reveals its critical role in health and disease, emphasizing the need for a holistic approach to health that considers the intricate interactions between our bodies and the microorganisms they host. Future research in microbiome science holds the potential to revolutionize medicine, offering new insights into disease prevention, diagnosis, and treatment. By understanding and harnessing the power of the microbiome, we can pave the way for innovative therapies and a deeper comprehension of human health and disease.

Proven Natural Remedies for Common Ailments

In our journey through the world of natural healing, it becomes clear that nature offers a bounty of remedies for the ailments that commonly afflict us. From the tension of headaches to the discomfort of digestive issues, natural remedies can provide relief with minimal side effects, aligning with the body's inherent processes. This chapter delves into a selection of proven natural remedies for some of the most common health concerns, guided by the wisdom and practices endorsed by Barbara O'Neill. Let's explore how simple, natural approaches can be powerful allies in restoring health and well-being.

Detailed Guide On Natural Remedies

Acne

A common skin condition, can be addressed through natural means focusing on internal health and external care:

- **Aloe Vera:** Known for its anti-inflammatory and healing properties, aloe vera gel can be applied directly to the skin to soothe and heal acne lesions.

- **Dietary Changes:** Reducing dairy and sugar intake can help manage acne, as both can contribute to inflammation and hormonal imbalances that trigger breakouts.

- **Tea Tree Oil:** A natural antiseptic, diluted tea tree oil can be applied to acne spots to reduce inflammation and bacteria.

What Barbara would say: *"Acne is not just a surface problem; it's a signal from your body that something is out of balance internally. It often stems from dietary triggers, hormonal imbalances, or a buildup of toxins. By adopting a clean, whole-foods diet and ensuring proper hydration, you can help your body detoxify and correct the imbalances contributing to acne. External treatments like aloe vera and tea tree oil can soothe and heal, but true healing starts from within."*

Anxiety

Anxiety affects many and can be alleviated through natural, calming practices:

- **Deep Breathing Exercises:** Practicing deep, controlled breathing can help reduce anxiety by calming the nervous system.

- **Herbal Teas:** Chamomile and green tea contain compounds that can help soothe anxiety and promote relaxation.

- **Physical Activity:** Regular exercise, especially outdoor activities like walking or gardening, can significantly reduce anxiety levels.

What Barbara would say: *"Anxiety is often a response to stress and can be exacerbated by our modern, fast-paced lifestyle. It's crucial to incorporate calming practices into your daily routine, such as deep breathing exercises, to help manage stress levels. Herbal teas and physical activity are nature's gifts for calming the mind and strengthening the body's resilience to stress. Remember, nurturing your mental and emotional well-being is just as important as taking care of your physical health."*

Eczema

Eczema, or atopic dermatitis, causes dry, itchy skin. Natural remedies focus on reducing inflammation and soothing the skin:

- **Coconut Oil:** Applying coconut oil to the affected areas can moisturize the skin and reduce eczema's itchiness and flaking.

- **Oatmeal Baths:** Colloidal oatmeal baths can soothe and protect irritated skin, providing relief from eczema symptoms.

- **Omega-3 Fatty Acids:** Increasing omega-3 intake through diet or supplements can help reduce inflammation associated with eczema.

What Barbara would say: *"Eczema is a sign of deeper inflammation within the body, often linked to diet and allergens. To address eczema, focus on anti-inflammatory foods and eliminate potential triggers like dairy or gluten. Topical remedies like coconut oil can provide relief, but healing eczema involves treating the whole person, not just the skin. Ensuring a balanced diet and managing stress are key steps toward soothing eczema from the inside out."*

Headaches

Headaches, whether tension-related or migraines, can significantly impact quality of life. Before reaching for over-the-counter pain relief, consider these natural alternatives:

- **Peppermint Oil:** Applied topically, peppermint oil can help soothe tension headaches. A small amount rubbed on the forehead and temples creates a cooling sensation, promoting muscle relaxation and easing pain.

- **Hydration:** Often, headaches are a sign of dehydration. Drinking water steadily throughout the day can prevent and alleviate headache symptoms.

- **Magnesium:** A natural muscle relaxant, magnesium can be particularly effective for migraines. Incorporating magnesium-rich foods like almonds, spinach, and bananas into your diet, or considering supplementation, may reduce headache frequency.

What Barbara would say: *"Headaches often signal dehydration, nutritional deficiencies, or tension. Before turning to pain medication, assess your hydration levels, diet, and stress factors. Natural remedies like peppermint oil can provide immediate relief, but preventing headaches also involves regular hydration, adequate magnesium intake, and techniques to manage stress effectively. Listen to your body—it's telling you it needs something."*

Digestive Issues

Digestive problems, including bloating, indigestion, and irritable bowel syndrome (IBS), can be both uncomfortable and disruptive. Nature provides several remedies to support digestive health:

- **Ginger:** Known for its anti-inflammatory and gastrointestinal soothing properties, ginger can alleviate nausea, bloating, and indigestion. A warm ginger tea can be particularly comforting.

- **Probiotics:** Maintaining a healthy gut flora is essential for digestive health. Probiotics, found in fermented foods like yogurt, kefir, and sauerkraut, can help balance the digestive system, easing symptoms of IBS and other digestive disorders.

- **Fiber:** A diet high in fiber from fruits, vegetables, and whole grains can improve digestion, prevent constipation, and maintain a healthy gut.

What Barbara would say: *"Digestive problems reflect how we nourish our bodies and manage stress. A diet rich in whole, plant-based foods and probiotics supports a healthy gut microbiome, crucial for digestion and overall health. Remember, your gut is your 'second brain,' and its well-being affects your entire body. Incorporating fiber, staying hydrated, and eating mindfully are practical steps to support digestive health."*

Sleep Issues

A good night's sleep is foundational to health, yet many people struggle with insomnia and restlessness. Natural remedies can help encourage a more restful sleep:

- **Lavender:** The scent of lavender has been shown to lower blood pressure and heart rate, creating a calming effect conducive to sleep. Consider lavender essential oil in a diffuser or a dried lavender sachet near your pillow.

- **Chamomile Tea:** Chamomile is a mild tranquilizer and sleep-inducer. Its calming effects may help improve sleep quality when consumed before bedtime.

- **Routine:** Establishing a calming pre-sleep routine, including activities like reading or a warm bath, can signal your body that it's time to wind down. Keeping electronics out of the bedroom can also improve sleep quality.

What Barbara would say: *"Sleep is foundational to health, yet often neglected in our busy lives. Creating a calming bedtime routine and optimizing your sleep environment can significantly improve sleep quality. Herbs like lavender and practices like magnesium supplementation can support relaxation. Remember, the quality of your sleep directly impacts your physical and mental health."*

Energy Levels

Maintaining steady energy levels can be a challenge in our busy lives. Natural remedies can help boost vitality without the crash associated with caffeine and sugar:

- **Ashwagandha:** An adaptogen, ashwagandha can help the body manage stress and improve energy levels. It can be taken as a supplement or found in some health foods.

- **B Vitamins:** Vital for energy production, B vitamins can be found in whole grains, meats, eggs, and greens. Consider a B-complex supplement if your diet may be lacking.

- **Hydration and Light Exercise:** Never underestimate the power of hydration and moderate exercise, like walking, to boost energy levels and improve overall well-being.

What Barbara would say: *"Low energy levels can be a symptom of nutritional deficiencies, dehydration, or inadequate rest. Natural adaptogens like ashwagandha and ensuring a diet rich in B vitamins can help boost your energy naturally. Also, never underestimate the power of hydration and regular, gentle exercise to invigorate the body and mind."*

Back Pain

Back pain, a common issue affecting many, can significantly impact daily activities. Natural remedies for back pain focus on reducing inflammation and improving mobility:

- **Heat Therapy:** Applying a hot water bottle or a heating pad to the affected area can help relax muscles and improve blood circulation, offering relief from pain.

- **Turmeric:** Known for its anti-inflammatory properties, turmeric can be consumed in food, as a tea, or as a supplement to help reduce inflammation and pain.

- **Yoga:** Gentle yoga poses can stretch and strengthen back muscles, improving posture and alleviating pain over time.

What Barbara would say: *"Back pain is often the result of poor posture, lack of physical activity, or stress. Incorporating gentle exercises and heat therapy can provide relief, but addressing the root cause is essential. Strengthening the core and maintaining flexibility through yoga or stretching exercises can help prevent future pain. Listen to your body and provide it with the movement and care it needs."*

Menstruation Ills

Menstrual cramps and other menstruation-related discomforts can be debilitating. Natural approaches aim to ease these symptoms:

Heat Application: Just as with back pain, applying heat to the lower abdomen can relax the muscles and ease menstrual cramps.

Chamomile Tea: Its antispasmodic properties can help reduce muscle spasms and serve as a natural pain reliever during menstruation.

Omega-3 Fatty Acids: Incorporating foods rich in omega-3s, such as fish, flaxseeds, and walnuts, or taking supplements, can help reduce the intensity of cramps.

What Barbara would say: *"Menstrual discomfort is influenced by diet, stress, and overall health. Natural heat application and omega-3 fatty acids can offer relief, but holistic management involves balancing hormones through proper nutrition and stress reduction. Understanding and working with your body's natural rhythms, rather than against them, can alleviate menstruation ills."*

Joint Pain

Natural remedies for joint pain aim to reduce inflammation and improve joint health:

- **Turmeric and Ginger Tea:** Both turmeric and ginger have anti-inflammatory properties, making a combined tea an effective remedy for reducing joint pain.

- **Epsom Salt Baths:** Soaking in a bath with Epsom salts can help relieve joint pain and muscle soreness through the skin's absorption of magnesium.

- **Exercise:** Low-impact exercises, such as swimming or cycling, can strengthen the muscles around the joints, providing support and reducing pain.

Toothache

Toothaches can be agonizing, stemming from various causes like decay, infection, or injury. While severe cases should be seen by a dentist, some natural remedies can provide temporary relief:

Clove Oil: With its numbing effect, clove oil can be applied to the affected tooth or gum area to alleviate pain. A drop of oil on a cotton ball placed gently on the sore spot works effectively.

Salt Water Rinse: A saltwater rinse can help reduce inflammation and kill bacteria in the mouth. Dissolve a teaspoon of salt in a cup of warm water and use it as a mouth rinse.

Garlic: Known for its antibacterial properties, a paste of crushed garlic applied to the tooth or chewing a clove of garlic can provide relief.

What Barbara would say: *"A toothache is a clear signal from your body that oral health cannot be ignored. While remedies like clove oil provide temporary relief, addressing dietary habits and ensuring proper oral hygiene are crucial for long-term health. A diet low in sugar and rich in minerals supports strong teeth and gums. Remember, oral health is a window to your overall health."*

Natural Remedies for Various Health Conditions

This chapter delves into the art and science of natural remedies, showcasing the healing powers of simple ingredients like castor oil, onions, garlic, ginger, potatoes, cayenne pepper, and charcoal. Each of these natural elements offers unique properties that can address a wide range of health conditions, from the common cold to more complex issues like cysts and inflammation.

Castor Oil Compresses: The therapeutic use of castor oil compresses is a testament to the profound impact that natural remedies can have on our health. Known for their deep penetration, castor oil compresses are adept at breaking up lumps, bumps, and adhesions. Conditions such as cysts, breast cancer, irritable bowel syndrome, constipation, gallbladder stones, and bone spurs can all benefit from this simple yet effective treatment. The method involves creating a thick pack using an incontinence pad or cloth, soaked in castor oil, and secured with masking tape to ensure the oil stays in contact with the skin for optimal effect.

Onion Poultices; The humble onion, with its potent medicinal properties, serves as a versatile remedy for a variety of ailments. Cooked onions, applied warm, can draw out infections and ease the pain of earaches and boils. Conversely, raw onions, when sliced and wrapped in cloth, can soothe sore throats and, intriguingly, treat coughs when placed on the bottom of the feet overnight. The chapter also introduces a simple yet effective onion cough syrup, layering chopped onions and honey to create a powerful remedy for respiratory issues.

Garlic for Immune Support: Garlic's reputation as a powerful antimicrobial agent is well-deserved. Its antiviral, antibacterial, and antifungal properties make it a cornerstone of immune support. Consuming raw garlic cloves or incorporating them into a "flu bomb" concoction with ginger, eucalyptus oil, cayenne pepper, lemon juice, and honey can offer a potent defense against flu symptoms. Additionally, the traditional practice of applying garlic slices to the feet underscores garlic's role in boosting the body's immune response.

Ginger Poultices: Ginger, celebrated for its anti-inflammatory properties, is particularly effective in poultice form for treating inflamed joints. The warmth and healing compounds of ginger can significantly alleviate the pain and inflammation associated with arthritis or gout. The preparation and application of a ginger poultice highlight its therapeutic potential, offering relief and comfort to those suffering from joint pain.

Potato Poultices: Potato poultices embody the gentle, cooling relief that natural remedies can provide. Recommended for tissue inflammation, such as swollen eyes, ingrown toenails, and splinters, potatoes can draw out infection and reduce swelling effectively. The anecdotal evidence shared in this chapter illustrates the poultice's soothing capabilities, offering a testament to the potato's understated healing power.

Cayenne Pepper: Cayenne pepper's role in stimulating blood flow and improving circulation is unparalleled. Its ability to thin blood, strengthen arterial walls, and open capillaries makes it a versatile remedy. Whether used internally to aid digestion or externally in compresses to warm cold feet and enhance blood flow, cayenne pepper exemplifies the dynamic healing potential of natural ingredients.

Charcoal Poultices: Concluding this exploration of natural remedies is the discussion on charcoal's adsorptive power. Charcoal poultices bind toxins effectively, making them indispensable for treating bee stings, spider bites, and other conditions requiring toxin removal. The chapter provides a practical guide to creating a no-mess charcoal poultice with psyllium, ensuring easy and efficient application.

Each remedy presented in this chapter offers a glimpse into the vast potential of natural ingredients to heal and restore. As we navigate the complexities of health and wellness, these traditional remedies stand as beacons of hope, demonstrating that sometimes, the simplest solutions are the most profound. Embracing these natural remedies invites us to reconnect with the wisdom of the past, empowering us to take control of our health in the most natural way possible.

The Science Behind Natural Remedies

In exploring the realm of natural healing, the marriage of ancient wisdom with modern science unveils a powerful synergy. The evidence-based practices and research findings that support natural remedies not only validate their efficacy but also deepen our understanding of holistic health. As we delve into this rich terrain, let's keep our minds open and curious. *How do these natural practices stand up to the scrutiny of modern research? And what can this tell us about the path to optimal health?*

The world of natural healing is vast and varied, encompassing a wide range of practices from herbal remedies to dietary interventions. While skeptics often question their validity, a growing body of scientific research supports the effectiveness of many natural treatments. Let's explore some key findings.

Herbal Remedies: Herbal remedies have been used for centuries to treat a myriad of ailments. *But what does science say?* Take turmeric, for example, widely acclaimed for its anti-inflammatory properties. A study published in the Journal of Medicinal Food confirms that curcumin, the active compound in turmeric, effectively reduces inflammation in conditions like arthritis, supporting its traditional use. *And what about ginger for nausea?* Research in the European Journal of Gastroenterology & Hepatology shows that ginger is not only effective in alleviating post-operative nausea but also in reducing symptoms of morning sickness in pregnancy. *Isn't it fascinating to see how these ancient remedies hold up under the lens of modern research?*

Dietary Interventions: Dietary interventions are cornerstone practices in natural healing, advocating for whole, nutrient-dense foods to support health. *The evidence?* A systematic review in the American Journal of Clinical Nutrition highlights the role of Mediterranean diets in reducing the risk of cardiovascular diseases, showcasing the power of diet in preventive healthcare. Similarly, the impact of fiber on digestive health is well-documented, with studies indicating its role in reducing the incidence of colorectal cancer and improving gut microbiota.

Physical Activity and Mental Health: The connection between physical activity and mental health is another area where evidence aligns beautifully with natural healing principles. Research published in The Lancet Psychiatry journal found regular exercise to be significantly associated with reduced mental health burdens. Whether it's yoga, walking, or more vigorous exercise, the act of moving our bodies not only strengthens us physically but also elevates our mood and resilience.

Sleep Hygiene: Sleep hygiene practices, often recommended in natural healing, have a strong backing in research. Studies underscore the importance of regular sleep patterns and a conducive sleep environment for enhancing sleep quality and overall health. For instance, research in the Journal of Clinical Sleep Medicine highlights the negative impact of electronic device use before bedtime on sleep, reinforcing the advice to create tech-free sanctuaries for rest. *How might refining your sleep hygiene practices transform your well-being?*

As we navigate through these evidence-based practices and research findings, it's clear that the wisdom of natural healing and the rigor of scientific inquiry are not at odds but are, in fact, complementary. This fusion of knowledge empowers us to approach health holistically, with both reverence for tradition and respect for empirical evidence. In embracing natural remedies and holistic practices, we're not just following ancient wisdom but are also aligning with scientifically validated approaches to health and wellness. *How does this blend of old and new influence your perspective on natural healing? And more importantly, how might it inspire you to integrate these practices into your daily life for enhanced health and vitality?* As we continue this journey, remember that the pursuit of health is both a personal and a universal quest.

The evidence supports a holistic approach, emphasizing the interconnectedness of our physical, mental, and emotional well-being.

How To Prepare And Use These Remedies Safely

Navigating the path of natural remedies requires a harmonious blend of passion for nature's offerings and meticulous attention to safety protocols. The enchantment of harnessing nature's bounty for healing purposes is undeniably compelling. However, it's essential to remember that the natural world's gifts, while bountiful, demand respect and understanding to be used effectively and safely. The journey toward integrating natural remedies into our lives involves a dedicated exploration of dosages, quality, preparation, interactions, and an ongoing dialogue with our bodies and healthcare professionals.

Understanding Dosages: The effectiveness and safety of natural remedies hinge significantly on dosage accuracy. Turmeric and ginger, celebrated for their anti-inflammatory and digestive benefits, exemplify the need for dosage precision. Starting with modest amounts and adjusting based on individual tolerance and health objectives can mitigate potential adverse effects. This approach underscores the importance of consulting with healthcare professionals or trusted sources knowledgeable in herbal medicine. These consultations can illuminate the appropriate dosages that harmonize with specific health conditions, thereby enhancing both the efficacy and safety of natural remedies.

Quality and Purity: The quest for natural remedies is also a quest for purity and quality. The therapeutic potential of any herbal supplement or essential oil is inextricably linked to its quality. Products that have undergone rigorous testing for purity and are free from detrimental additives stand as pillars of effective natural healing. Certifications from independent bodies often serve as beacons of quality, guiding individuals toward safer choices. Engaging in diligent research and scrutinizing product labels for such certifications becomes a crucial step in selecting remedies that promise both healing and safety.

Preparation Methods: The preparation of natural remedies is an art and science that significantly influences their healing attributes. The meticulous brewing of ginger tea for digestive relief, for instance, requires precise steeping times to unleash its beneficial compounds optimally. Similarly, the application of topical solutions like aloe vera or lavender oil necessitates an understanding of proper dilution techniques to avoid irritation while maximizing therapeutic benefits. This attention to detail in preparation not only safeguards against potential harm but also ensures the maximum efficacy of the remedy.

Interaction Awareness: A critical aspect of safely incorporating natural remedies into health regimens is awareness of their potential interactions with medications, supplements, or other herbal treatments. The example of St. John's Wort illustrates the complexity of herbal interactions, necessitating thorough research and professional consultation prior to integration into one's health plan. This vigilance helps safeguard against unintended consequences and ensures that natural remedies complement rather than complicate health management strategies.

Listening to Your Body: The cornerstone of safely using natural remedies lies in attuning to one's body. The unique reactions and responses to different treatments underscore the importance of personal awareness and adaptability. Adjusting dosages or discontinuing use in response to adverse effects exemplifies the responsive and respectful approach required in natural healing. This personalized strategy emphasizes the body's role as the ultimate arbiter of what is beneficial or harmful.

Ongoing Education and Consultation: The dynamic landscape of natural healing, with its ever-expanding repository of knowledge and practices, calls for continuous learning and professional engagement. Staying abreast of the latest research and seeking guidance from healthcare practitioners skilled in both conventional and holistic medicine provides a foundation for informed and safe use of natural remedies. This educational commitment ensures that individuals are well-equipped to navigate the complexities of natural healing with confidence and discernment.

Nutrition and Detoxification According to Barbara O'Neill

Embarking on a journey of natural healing, guided by Barbara O'Neill's insights, transforms our approach to nutrition and detoxification into an empowering quest for vitality. O'Neill's perspective sheds light on how closely intertwined our eating habits are with our body's natural ability to heal and rejuvenate itself. Let's navigate this path with a fresh lens, focusing on making our diet a vibrant source of health and energy.

O'Neill's Dietary Recommendations for Optimal Health

Imagine walking through a lush garden or a vibrant farmer's market. This is where our journey begins. O'Neill encourages us to fill our baskets with a rainbow of fruits, vegetables, whole grains, nuts, and seeds. These aren't just foods; they're life forces, rich in the nutrients our bodies crave for optimal function. Integrating a variety of these whole foods into our diet not only supports our body's internal systems but also kickstarts the detoxification process, naturally eliminating toxins and bolstering our defenses against nutrient deficiencies.

Checklist for Embracing Whole Foods:

- **Fruits and Vegetables:** Aim for color and variety. Each color provides different antioxidants and phytonutrients.

- **Whole Grains**: Quinoa, barley, oats, and brown rice should be staples in your pantry.

- **Nuts and Seeds:** Almonds, walnuts, flaxseeds, and chia seeds offer essential fatty acids and proteins.

Transitioning towards a diet that celebrates plant-based foods isn't about strict dietary labels but embracing a lifestyle that prioritizes plants as the main act on your plate. This shift can significantly reduce inflammation and lower the risk of developing chronic diseases. *Have you noticed how your body feels after a meal rich in plants compared to one heavy in processed foods?*

Foods to Favor:

- **Legumes:** Beans, lentils, and chickpeas are excellent protein sources.

- **Leafy Greens:** Spinach, kale, and Swiss chard are nutrient powerhouses.

- **Whole Fruits:** Berries, apples, and bananas are nature's perfect snacks.

Embarking on a holistic health journey, we encounter the essence of vitality—water. Barbara O'Neill positions water as nature's most profound elixir, underscoring its pivotal role in hydrating our bodies and facilitating the natural detoxification process. Each sip of clean, filtered water or herbal tea we take acts as a vital supporter of our bodily functions, washing away toxins and nurturing every cell. *Reflect for a moment—how much water have you embraced today?* Integrating hydration into our daily lives isn't just a routine; it's a transformative ritual that enhances our well-being in untold ways.

Flowing seamlessly from the topic of hydration, we delve into the rejuvenating practice of fasting. Approached with intention and careful preparation, fasting offers our digestive systems a pause, a respite that empowers our bodies to focus inward on healing and purging toxins. This ancient practice, revived and refined through O'Neill's guidance, isn't about deprivation but renewal. Listening to our body's cues during fasting reveals when and how this practice can serve as a potent tool for detoxification and rejuvenation, aligning with our body's natural rhythms and needs. Yet, as we hydrate and fast, another crucial element in our health odyssey is minimizing toxin exposure—a task as critical as the nutrients we consciously consume. O'Neill urges us to make thoughtful choices, opting for organic produce over conventionally grown counterparts laden with pesticides and to sidestep processed foods in favor of nature's bounty. This conscious selection significantly reduces the toxic burden our bodies contend with, facilitating a more efficient detoxification process. *Have you pondered the impact of your food choices on your body's ability to cleanse and renew?*

Recognizing our individuality, O'Neill champions a personalized nutrition strategy, asserting that a one-size-fits-all approach falls short of meeting our unique health requirements. Tailoring our diet to reflect our personal health status, lifestyle, and specific nutritional needs elevates the journey from mere sustenance to a targeted, healing crusade. Engaging with healthcare professionals to customize our dietary choices enhances this personalization, ensuring our path to wellness is as unique as our DNA.

In integrating these principles into our lives, we not only fuel our bodies with the essence of natural vitality but also align our eating habits with a deeper, more holistic understanding of health. This isn't just about avoiding illness; it's about thriving. As we adopt Barbara O'Neill's holistic strategies for nutrition and detoxification, we empower ourselves to live in harmony with our body's natural rhythms, embracing a life of wellness and vitality. *How will you begin to incorporate these changes into your daily routine, transforming your approach to health and wellness?*

Alkaline and Acid-Forming Foods

The foods we choose to consume play a leading role in scripting our health's narrative. Each bite, each morsel we ingest, acts not just as sustenance but as a potent signal to our body, influencing its internal environment and, by extension, its potential for disease or wellness. Understanding the intricate dance between alkaline and acid-forming foods is essential for maintaining our body's optimal health. This balance is not just a dietary choice; it's a foundation for preventing disease and fostering vitality. Let's delve into the pivotal role of pH balance in our health, the distinction between alkaline and acid-forming foods, and practical dietary recommendations to harness the power of food for wellness.

Our body is a finely tuned system that thrives within a specific pH range. The term "pH" stands for *"potential of hydrogen,"* a measure of the acidity or alkalinity of our body's fluids and tissues. This scale ranges from 0 to 14, with 7 being neutral. Below 7 indicates acidity, and above 7 signifies alkalinity. The human blood maintains a slightly alkaline pH of 7.35 to 7.45, essential for sustaining life. Cells, however, operate best at a slightly acidic pH of around 6.5, which is crucial for facilitating the myriad of chemical reactions necessary for proper cellular function.

Alkaline-Forming Foods: These foods play a critical role in promoting health by helping to maintain an optimal pH balance in the body. Despite their initial acidity, foods like lemons and other citrus fruits become alkaline during the digestive process. Dark green leafy vegetables, along with a variety of other vegetables, grains like millet, quinoa, amaranth, spelt, and kamut, as well as almonds, Brazil nuts, and seeds, are rich in alkaline minerals such as sodium, potassium, calcium, magnesium, and iron. These foods contribute to creating an alkaline environment that supports cellular health and overall well-being.

Acid-Forming Foods: Conversely, acid-forming foods can disrupt our body's pH balance, contributing to an acidic environment that may encourage disease progression. Common acid-forming foods include meat, refined sugars, hybridized wheat, aged cheeses, caffeine, alcohol, and tobacco. These items are high in acid-forming minerals like phosphorus, sulfur, and chlorine, which can challenge the body's ability to maintain its delicate pH balance.

The concept that diet can significantly impact our risk of developing diseases, particularly those as formidable as cancer, is both a cautionary tale and a beacon of hope. Cancer cells, as we've come to understand, thrive in environments characterized by low oxygen levels and an abundance of sugar—a scenario unfortunately promoted by a diet heavy in acid-forming foods. Conversely, an alkaline diet, abundant in nutrients and conducive to higher oxygen availability, erects a formidable barrier against the incursion of disease, fortifying the body's natural defenses. This dialogue between our dietary choices and our body's health extends beyond the food itself to encompass the very essence of life—water. Hydration, or the lack thereof, plays a pivotal role in maintaining the delicate balance of our body's pH level. The kidneys, those unsung heroes of homeostasis, rely on adequate hydration to perform their critical function of regulating blood pH. Through the excretion of excess acids or bases, they ensure that our internal environment remains within the narrow confines conducive to life. Thus, our water intake becomes a key player in the detoxification process, aiding the kidneys in their ceaseless task and supporting overall health.

However, the narrative of diet is as varied and complex as the individuals it affects. This is exemplified in the discussion of **nightshade vegetables**—*tomatoes, bell peppers, eggplants, and potatoes*—which, despite their nutritional benefits, may not agree with everyone. For some, these vegetables can incite inflammation, underscoring the critical importance of personalized nutrition. This concept of individuality in dietary needs highlights a fundamental truth: what nourishes one body might not suit another. Recognizing and respecting our unique responses to certain foods is crucial in tailoring a diet that not only nourishes but also protects. Navigating this complex landscape of dietary choices, Barbara O'Neill offers sage advice: *a balanced diet comprising mainly alkaline-forming foods, with a smaller proportion of acid-forming foods, can provide the foundation for robust health.* This balance is not about strict adherence to rigid dietary rules but about understanding and applying principles that support the body's natural functions, preventing disease before it takes root.

Weight Loss Made Easy

Embarking on a weight loss journey transcends the simplistic view of cutting calories and ramping up exercise routines. It's about nurturing a harmonious relationship with our bodies, understanding the profound impact of our dietary choices, and aligning our lifestyle with natural rhythms that promote health and vitality. Drawing upon a holistic approach to wellness, this chapter offers an empathetic guide to shedding excess weight through balanced nutrition, mindful meal timing, and integrating physical activity that resonates with the body's innate wisdom.

- **The Balanced Path to Nutrition:** Modern diet, abundant in high-carbohydrate foods such as bread, cereal, pasta, and sugars, significantly contributes to weight gain by providing more glucose than the body can efficiently use, leading to fat accumulation. A shift towards a diet low in refined carbohydrates and rich in fiber, moderate in proteins—preferably from plant sources—and abundant in healthy fats, marks the cornerstone of effective weight management. This balanced approach not only aids in reducing body fat but also supports overall health by ensuring that our meals are nutrient-dense and aligned with our body's needs.

- **Harnessing the Power of Meal Timing:** Our bodies operate on natural rhythms, and aligning our eating patterns with these rhythms can significantly enhance metabolism and facilitate weight loss. Consuming the majority of our calories earlier in the day, when our metabolic rate is higher, and reducing intake by evening, supports our body's natural processing of food. Furthermore, the concept of "time-restricted eating," which narrows eating windows to certain hours of the day, can further support weight management efforts by synchronizing meal times with our body's internal clock, promoting more efficient energy use and fat burning.

- **Hydration and the Role of Salt:** Adequate hydration is a key yet often overlooked component of weight loss. Drinking sufficient water throughout the day aids in maintaining metabolic balance and supports the body's natural detoxification processes. Coupled with the mindful consumption of whole salt, which provides essential minerals and aids in fluid balance, hydration becomes a simple yet effective tool in enhancing weight loss efforts.

- **The Vital Role of Exercise:** High-Intensity Interval Training (HIIT) is highlighted for its efficiency in burning fat and improving overall fitness within a condensed timeframe. By engaging in short bursts of intense activity followed by recovery periods, HIIT stimulates cellular processes that enhance fat burning and muscle preservation. This form of exercise is particularly effective due to its ability to increase the conversion of lactic acid and stimulate the production of the human growth hormone, key factors in weight loss and maintaining muscle mass.

- **Mind, Hormones, and Breath:** The journey to weight loss is as much mental as it is physical. Envisioning oneself achieving their weight loss goals can significantly impact success. Additionally, addressing hormonal imbalances plays a crucial role in managing weight. Strategies to balance hormones, particularly to manage excess estrogen, are essential components of a comprehensive weight loss plan.

Moreover, adopting proper breathing techniques, especially during exercise, can enhance oxygen delivery to tissues and promote relaxation, supporting the body's natural weight regulation mechanisms.

In conclusion, weight loss involves nurturing a deep, respectful partnership with our bodies, understanding the nutritional, physical, and psychological aspects that contribute to weight gain, and addressing these with patience, knowledge, and care. By adopting a balanced diet, aligning our eating patterns with our body's rhythms, staying hydrated, engaging in effective exercise, and attending to our hormonal and mental well-being, we embark on a path not just to weight loss, but to lasting health and vitality. This holistic approach, inspired by the wisdom of natural healing, offers a compassionate and sustainable path to achieving and maintaining a healthy weight.

The Power of Water Therapy

This elixir of life, so often taken for granted, holds the key to vitality, serving as the cornerstone of our physical and mental well-being. The human body, a marvel of biological engineering, can sustain itself for weeks without food, yet mere days without water underscore its critical importance. Proper hydration goes beyond quenching thirst; it's a vital practice for maintaining health and preventing a myriad of diseases.

The role of minerals in hydration, particularly sodium and potassium, is a tale of balance and harmony. Sodium, especially when sourced from natural reserves like Celtic or Himalayan salt, plays a crucial role in nutrient transport and cellular hydration. Unlike its heavily processed counterpart, table salt, these natural salts come replete with a spectrum of trace minerals. They facilitate the passage of water into cells, ensuring that each cell functions optimally. Barbara O'Neill's endorsement of Celtic or Himalayan salt over table salt stems from an understanding of these health benefits, coupled with a concern for the potential risks associated with the latter's consumption. Potassium, abundant in fruits and vegetables, is the unsung hero of cellular function. It works in concert with sodium, maintaining the delicate balance of cellular hydration and function. This interplay is essential for a host of bodily processes, from nerve signal transmission to muscle contraction and heart function.

The impact of hydration extends its reach across various aspects of health, influencing digestion, blood pressure regulation, brain function, and joint health. Conversely, dehydration casts a long shadow, leading to headaches, back pain, cognitive impairments, and more. Such ailments serve as a clarion call, reminding us of water's pivotal role in our health ecosystem. Barbara O'Neill's recommendation to consume at least eight glasses of water daily, with adjustments for physical activity and environmental conditions, is more than a guideline; it's a lifeline. She advocates for a consistent, mindful approach to hydration—drinking water in small, frequent amounts throughout the day to optimize absorption and utilization. To navigate the path to optimal hydration, practical tips abound. Starting the day with water, possibly with a pinch of Celtic salt to enhance absorption, sets a positive tone for hydration practices. Ensuring a balanced intake of minerals through a diet rich in fruits, vegetables, and unrefined salts can fortify this foundation, promoting a state of well-being that permeates every cell.

What to Know About Fats

In a nutritional landscape often clouded by misinformation and oversimplified advice, Barbara sheds light on the complex and essential world of dietary fats. Her insights navigate the intricacies of essential fatty acids, debunk common myths about fats, and illuminate the path to understanding which fats nourish our bodies and which do harm. At the heart of O'Neill's philosophy is the distinction between essential fatty acids: **omega-3 and omega-6.** These building blocks of cellular health, with their characteristic double bonds, are indispensable for the fluidity and functionality of cell membranes. Their contribution spans a broad spectrum, from fostering brain health to mitigating inflammation. Yet, these essential nutrients are beyond our body's manufacturing capabilities, casting a spotlight on the importance of dietary sources.

Dispelling the myth that omega-3s are found predominantly in fish, Barbara turns our attention to the plant kingdom. Flaxseed and chia seeds emerge as potent sources of **alpha-linolenic acid (ALA)**, challenging preconceived notions and broadening our horizon towards plant-based nutrition. This revelation is not merely about dietary diversity; it underscores a fundamental principle of consuming nutrients in their most unadulterated form. The narrative deepens with the exploration of the body's capacity to convert ALA into the vital fatty acids **EPA** and **DHA**, essential for cell membrane repair and overall function. This natural alchemy within our bodies highlights the profound interconnectedness of nature and human biology, where plant-based omega-3s are transformed into complex fatty acids, pivotal for our well-being.

Yet, the integrity of these fats is precarious, vulnerable to the assaults of cooking and processing. Barbara cautions against the altered structures of processed oils and fats, advocating for a return to natural, whole sources. This call to action is not just a dietary recommendation; it's a plea for mindfulness in our consumption habits, recognizing the profound impact of these choices on our health. In this context, coconut oil stands as a paragon of healthy fats, challenging the stigma associated with saturated fats. Its medium-chain fatty acids, metabolized efficiently by the liver, exemplify the nuanced nature of fats, where certain saturated fats defy conventional wisdom and contribute positively to our health. This nuanced understanding extends to the broader category of saturated fats, inviting a reevaluation of their role in our diet. O'Neill's discourse on the matter is a clarion call to distinguish between natural sources of saturated fats and their chemically altered counterparts, highlighting the need for a balanced and informed approach.

The dangers of trans fats and hydrogenated oils are starkly outlined, with O'Neill warning against their profound health risks. This cautionary tale reinforces the importance of natural, unprocessed fats, advocating for a diet that embraces the diversity and richness of whole foods. O'Neill's holistic approach to diet, integrating natural fats with a bounty of vegetables, fruits, and whole grains, is a testament to her philosophy of nourishment. This balanced strategy is not just about physical health; it's a comprehensive approach to well-being, emphasizing the synergy between different nutrients and the importance of dietary harmony. Through O'Neill's lens, the world of dietary fats is demystified, transformed from a source of confusion into a landscape of opportunity. Her teachings offer not just dietary guidelines but a philosophy of nourishment, inviting us to embrace the complexity of fats with knowledge and grace. This chapter is more than a guide; it's an invitation to journey towards a healthier, more vibrant life, guided by the wisdom of understanding and choosing the right fats. In this narrative, fats are not foes but allies, essential components of a diet that nourishes, heals, and sustains.

Detoxification Practices

As we continue our holistic health journey, we arrive at the pivotal practice of detoxification. This process, intricately woven into Barbara O'Neill's philosophy, is not merely about eliminating toxins but about revitalizing our entire being. Detoxification practices, ranging from simple dietary adjustments to more structured cleansing routines, serve as bridges, reconnecting us with our body's innate capacity for self-renewal and healing.

Detoxification is the body's natural process of neutralizing and eliminating toxins, a critical function for maintaining health and vitality. O'Neill emphasizes that while our bodies are remarkably equipped for this task, the overwhelming presence of pollutants in our environment, food, and lifestyle can impede this intrinsic ability. Herein lies the beauty of intentional detox practices—they support the body's efforts, enhancing its natural cleansing processes. Engaging in detoxification practices offers a myriad of benefits, rejuvenating not just the physical body but also our mental and emotional landscapes. Here are some transformative advantages:

- **Enhanced Energy Levels:** As toxins are removed, our bodies function more efficiently, leading to an increase in energy and vitality. Imagine waking up feeling refreshed and invigorated, ready to embrace the day with open arms.

- **Improved Digestive Health:** Detox practices often involve dietary changes that promote gut health, leading to improved digestion and absorption of nutrients. It's like setting the reset button on your digestive system, allowing it to function at its peak.

- **Boosted Immune System:** By reducing the toxin load, our bodies can focus more on immune function, better equipping us to fend off illness. Think of it as fortifying your body's natural defenses, creating a shield against diseases.

- **Mental Clarity:** The clarity of mind that follows detoxification is akin to lifting a fog, enhancing focus and cognitive function. It's as if your brain is getting a breath of fresh air, allowing for clearer thought and concentration.

- **Emotional Balance:** The process of detoxification can also lead to emotional cleansing, releasing stored emotions and fostering a sense of well-being. It's an opportunity for emotional renewal, paving the way for a more balanced and harmonious state of mind.

O'Neill advocates for various accessible and effective detoxification practices, emphasizing the importance of choosing methods that resonate with your body and lifestyle. Some of these practices include:

- **Dietary Adjustments:** Incorporating detoxifying foods like leafy greens, berries, and garlic into your diet supports the body's cleansing processes.

- **Hydration:** Continuing to prioritize hydration, with an emphasis on clean water and herbal teas, aids in flushing toxins from the body.

- **Fasting and Intermittent Fasting:** These practices give the digestive system a break, promoting healing and toxin elimination.

- **Exercise:** Regular physical activity, especially sweating through exercise, helps expel toxins through the skin.

- **Mindfulness and Stress Reduction:** Techniques such as meditation and yoga support emotional detoxification, reducing the impact of stress on physical health.

By integrating these detoxification practices into our daily routines, we not only support our body's natural cleansing mechanisms but also pave the way for a holistic transformation. This journey through detoxification, guided by Barbara O'Neill's wisdom, is a testament to the profound interconnectedness of our physical, mental, and emotional health. As we embrace these practices, we unlock the door to a revitalized, balanced, and deeply nourished existence, reaffirming our commitment to a life of wellness and harmony. But hold on a moment, I can hear you thinking: *"Yeah, great, but how on earth do I integrate all this great advice into my busy routine?"*

Creating a practical action plan that blends Barbara O'Neill's detoxification practices into a weekly routine can make a significant difference, even for those with the busiest of schedules. The key is to integrate small, manageable habits that collectively contribute to a powerful detoxification process. Here's how you can incorporate dietary adjustments, hydration, fasting, exercise, and mindfulness into your week for an effective detox. Here is an easily actionable example:

Monday: Kickstart with Hydration and Light Exercise

- Morning: Begin your day with a glass of warm lemon water to stimulate digestion and hydration.

- Daytime: Carry a reusable water bottle and aim for at least 2 liters of water throughout the day, infusing it with slices of cucumber or berries for an antioxidant boost.

- Evening: Engage in a 30-minute brisk walk or a gentle yoga session to encourage circulation and sweating, followed by a mindfulness meditation before bed.

Tuesday: Focus on Dietary Adjustments

- Morning: Opt for a smoothie packed with leafy greens, berries, and a teaspoon of ground flaxseed to fuel your body with detoxifying nutrients.

- Lunch and Dinner: Incorporate a salad rich in mixed greens, vegetables, and a garlic-based dressing. Choose whole grains like quinoa or brown rice as sides.

- Snacks: Reach for fresh fruit or a small handful of nuts to keep energy levels steady.

Wednesday: Introduce Intermittent Fasting

- Morning to Afternoon: If new to fasting, start with a 14-hour window, including sleep time. Skip breakfast and drink herbal teas or water to support hydration.

- Lunch: Break your fast with a balanced meal focusing on vegetables, lean protein, and healthy fats.

- Evening: Ensure your last meal is before 7 PM to maintain the fasting window, and include mindfulness practices to enhance stress reduction.

Thursday: Hydrate and Reflect

- All Day: Focus intensively on hydration, aiming for 3 liters of water and herbal tea. Reflect on any changes in how you feel with increased fluid intake.

- Evening: Dedicate time to journaling or a meditative practice to reflect on your week's progress, noting any shifts in your physical or emotional state.

Friday: Active Detox Day

- Morning: Start with dynamic stretching or a light jog to boost detoxification through sweat.

- Daytime: Continue with your dietary adjustments, incorporating detoxifying foods into all meals.

- Evening: Attend a yoga or fitness class that encourages detoxification through movement, like a hot yoga session.

Saturday: Social Detox and Relaxation

- Daytime: Engage in social activities that promote well-being, such as a nature hike with friends or family. Pack a picnic with detox-friendly foods.

- Evening: Treat yourself to a relaxing bath with Epsom salts to support detoxification and muscle relaxation, followed by an early night to promote restorative sleep.

Sunday: Reflective Fasting and Planning

- Morning: Engage in another round of intermittent fasting, using this time to plan your meals and activities for the coming week.

- Afternoon: Break your fast with a nutritious meal, and spend some time in meal prep for the week, focusing on incorporating a variety of detoxifying foods.

- Evening: Close your week with a gentle yoga session and meditation, setting intentions for the week ahead.

This weekly plan illustrates that incorporating detoxification practices into a busy lifestyle is both achievable and beneficial. It's about making intentional choices that align with your health goals, using Barbara O'Neill's principles as a guide to nurture and rejuvenate your body through thoughtful nutrition, hydration, physical activity, and mindfulness practices.

Planning a Balanced Diet

Crafting a balanced, nutritious diet that aligns with Barbara O'Neill's teachings involves a harmonious blend of whole foods, hydration, and mindful eating practices. O'Neill's approach is not just about what we eat but how we eat, emphasizing the importance of nourishing the body with foods that support its natural detoxification and healing processes. Here's how you can plan a week of meals and habits that resonate with this holistic philosophy, ensuring that your diet is not only balanced and nutritious but also sustainable and enriching. Before diving into meal planning, it's crucial to grasp the core components of a diet inspired by O'Neill's teachings:

- Whole Foods: Focus on fruits, vegetables, whole grains, nuts, seeds, and legumes.

- Plant-based Predominance: While not exclusively vegetarian, the diet leans heavily on plant-based foods for their nutrients, fiber, and antioxidants.

- Hydration: Adequate water intake is essential for digestion, detoxification, and overall vitality.

- Mindful Eating: Pay attention to your body's hunger and fullness cues, eating slowly and appreciatively.

Weekly Meal Planning Guide

Monday: Detox Focus

- Breakfast: Smoothie with spinach, banana, blueberries, flaxseed, and almond milk.

- Lunch: Quinoa salad with mixed greens, cherry tomatoes, cucumber, avocado, and lemon-tahini dressing.

- Dinner: Baked sweet potato, steamed broccoli, and grilled tofu with a ginger-garlic sauce.

- Hydration: Start the day with warm lemon water and aim for 2-3 liters of water throughout the day.

Tuesday: High Fiber

- Breakfast: Oatmeal topped with sliced apples, walnuts, and a dash of cinnamon.

- Lunch: Lentil soup with a side of mixed greens salad and whole-grain bread.

- Dinner: Stir-fried vegetables (bell peppers, snap peas, carrots) with tempeh over brown rice.

- Snack: Fresh fruit or vegetable sticks with hummus.

Wednesday: Plant Protein Boost

- Breakfast: Chia pudding made with coconut milk and topped with mixed berries.

- Lunch: Chickpea and avocado wrap with spinach and sprouts.

- Dinner: Black bean tacos with corn tortillas, salsa, lettuce, and cashew cheese.

- Snack: A handful of almonds or a protein-rich smoothie.

Thursday: Hydration & Light Meals

- Breakfast: Fruit salad with a drizzle of lemon juice and a sprinkle of chia seeds.

- Lunch: Gazpacho soup with a side quinoa tabbouleh.

- Dinner: Baked salmon with a side of steamed asparagus and wild rice.

- Hydration: Herbal teas and infused waters throughout the day.

Friday: Omega-3 Fatty Acids

- Breakfast: Flaxseed meal and almond flour pancakes with a side of mixed berries.

- Lunch: Salad with spinach, walnuts, sliced pear, and flaked salmon.

- Dinner: Grilled mackerel with a side of roasted Brussels sprouts and sweet potato mash.

- Snack: A small serving of dark chocolate or avocado slices.

Saturday: Colorful Variety

- Breakfast: Vegetable omelet with a side of whole-grain toast and avocado.

- Lunch: Buddha bowl with quinoa, beets, carrots, kale, and tahini dressing.

- Dinner: Ratatouille served over a bed of whole-grain pasta.

- Snack: Freshly squeezed juice or a piece of fruit.

Sunday: Mindful Eating Practice

- Breakfast: Green tea and a bowl of mixed fruit, eaten slowly and mindfully.

- Lunch: Roasted vegetable and hummus sandwich on whole-grain bread.

- Dinner: Grilled portobello mushrooms with herbed quinoa and a side salad.

- Snack: Medjool dates or a homemade granola bar.

By planning your meals with intention and mindfulness, you're not just feeding your body; you're nurturing your soul. This balanced, nutritious diet is designed to support your body's needs, promoting detoxification, healing, and overall well-being. Remember, the journey to health is personal and evolving—embrace the flexibility and joy in nourishing yourself well.

Caring for Your System- A Holistic Journey

The Gut Health

In the grand orchestra of the human body, where each organ and process contributes its unique melody, the gut conducts a symphony central to our health and vitality. This section, based on Barbara O'Neill's profound insights, invites us on a holistic journey through the digestive system, revealing the nuanced interplay of functions that sustain us. From the act of chewing to the final stages of absorption and elimination, we explore the pivotal roles of various digestive organs and the profound impact of our lifestyle choices on gut health.

Chewing and Its Significance

Imagine the act of chewing not just as a mechanical necessity but as the opening overture to the symphony of digestion. Within this seemingly mundane act lies the key to unlocking the full potential of our digestive capabilities. As we take the first bite, enzymes like amylase leap into action, initiating the breakdown of starches, setting the stage for the complex digestive process that follows. This moment, where food and enzyme meet, serves as a poignant reminder of the power of mindfulness in eating. Barbara O'Neill implores us to embrace the art of slow, intentional mastication, highlighting how such a simple act can significantly enhance the effectiveness of our digestion. Through this lens, chewing becomes more than just the first step in digestion—it's a ritual that honors the food we eat and the body that nourishes us, reminding us of the importance of being fully present with every bite.

The Stomach: A Crucible of Digestion

As we journey deeper into the digestive process, descending into the realm of the stomach, we are met with a scene of acidic splendor. Here, in this chamber of chemical transformation, proteins are meticulously dismantled by the enzyme pepsin, while hydrochloric acid stands guard, neutralizing potential pathogens that dare enter this sanctum. This acidic environment, far from being a mere byproduct of digestion, is foundational for nutrient absorption and the prevention of bacterial overgrowth. O'Neill elucidates the stomach's indispensable role in our digestive well-being, painting a picture of a body designed with innate wisdom to safeguard our health from the outset of digestion. The stomach's function is emblematic of the body's broader capabilities, a testament to the intricate design that supports life at every turn.

The Small Intestine: A Collaborative Effort

Venturing further into the depths of our digestive tract, we arrive at the small intestine, a site of remarkable collaboration among organs. In the duodenum, the first segment of the small intestine, a concerted effort unfolds as bile from the gallbladder and enzymes from the pancreas join forces, continuing the intricate dance of digesting fats and starches. This segment of our journey is marked by the presence of villi, tiny finger-like projections that line the walls of the small intestine, where the final act of nutrient absorption takes place. These villi, supported by a diverse and balanced gut flora, serve as the gatekeepers for nutrients entering our bloodstream, facilitating a transfer that is essential for our nourishment and vitality. O'Neill emphasizes the interconnectedness of our body's systems here, showcasing the delicate balance and cooperation needed to sustain life. The small intestine, with its complex ecosystem of microbes and enzymes, stands as a microcosm of the broader narrative of digestion—a tale of unity and symbiosis that underscores the holistic nature of our health.

The Colon: Guardian of Water and Nutrients

Our exploration continues with the colon, a vital organ responsible for water reabsorption, stool formation, and the final stages of nutrient absorption. Here, dietary fiber shines as a hero, ensuring regular bowel movements and acting as a bulwark against constipation. Beyond its functional role, fiber serves as a prebiotic, fostering a thriving ecosystem of gut flora essential for optimal health. Contrary to outdated notions, the appendix is unveiled as a crucial ally, supporting our immune system and maintaining a healthy balance of gut bacteria. This reevaluation of the appendix's role invites us to appreciate the complexity and interconnectedness of our digestive system.

Key Takeaways

Barbara O'Neill emphasizes the critical influence of diet on gastrointestinal well-being, painting a vivid picture of how modern dietary pitfalls disrupt our digestive equilibrium. Processed foods and excessive consumption of meat, dairy, and refined sugars not only challenge our gut's resilience but also predispose us to a spectrum of disorders. This narrative is not merely a critique but a clarion call to embrace whole, unprocessed foods. By advocating for dietary choices that align with our body's natural needs, O'Neill guides us toward a path of digestive harmony and overall health. This section is enriched with practical examples, illustrating how simple dietary adjustments can have profound impacts on our gut health. In a nod to both practicality and ancestral wisdom, our discussion culminates with the topic of correct toilet posture. The adoption of a squatting position, facilitated by modern aids like the "Squatty Potty," is more than a mere recommendation—it's an invitation to realign our habits with the body's natural design. This practice, simple yet transformative, exemplifies the fusion of traditional knowledge and contemporary convenience, offering a tangible step toward enhancing colon health.

Liver Health: The Cornerstone of Vitality

In the complex ecosystem that is the human body, the liver could be likened to a project manager given the multiplicity and significance of its functions. In this chapter, you will learn about the multifaceted roles the liver plays, its remarkable regenerative abilities, the profound impact our modern-day dietary and lifestyle habits have on its function, and what you can do, holistically, to maintain optimal health. The liver is often likened to a project manager because it regulates — comprehensively — our body's metabolic processes, including detoxification, metabolism (both fat and sugar), and the processing of nutrients. It's a good analogy in that it may help to better understand and appreciate the critical role the liver plays in maintaining the delicate balance of our body's health. Its functions go way beyond filtration — it is a multi-tasker, acting as a chemical factory converting the nutrients in our diets into forms our bodies can use, neutralizing toxins for excretion, and storing nutrients such as glycogen. So, in other words, maintaining optimal liver health is indispensable for overall well-being.

The Miracle of Regeneration

Among the liver's most awe-inspiring attributes is its unparalleled ability to regenerate and repair itself, a feature that sets it apart from other organs. This regenerative prowess is not just a biological curiosity; it embodies the liver's resilience and underscores the body's remarkable capacity for recovery and healing. Whether recovering from injury or compensating for damage, the liver's ability to regrow and restore itself serves as a powerful reminder of the body's inherent potential for self-healing, given the appropriate support and conditions. The seismic shift in dietary landscapes poses a formidable challenge to liver health. The prevalent high carbohydrate diets, saturated with glucose, exert undue pressure on liver function, leading to the accumulation of fat and spawning a host of metabolic disorders, including obesity and diabetes. This dietary conundrum highlights a dissonance between contemporary eating patterns and the nutritional sustenance our livers require, urging a reevaluation of our food choices in favor of liver health and metabolic harmony.

Detoxification: The Liver's Masterstroke

At the heart of the liver's myriad functions is its role in detoxification—a sophisticated process that transforms fat-soluble toxins into water-soluble forms for elimination. This critical function is essential for purging environmental toxins, safeguarding the body from potential harm. The liver's ability to neutralize and expel toxins is emblematic of the body's innate defense mechanisms, reflecting an evolutionary adaptation to protect against the diverse array of toxic challenges encountered in both natural and man-made environments. The liver's detoxification journey is intricately linked with a spectrum of nutrients. Antioxidants, such as beta carotene, vitamin C, and vitamin E, along with minerals and B vitamins, play pivotal roles in supporting liver function. Proteins, in particular, are indispensable in the second phase of detoxification, aiding in the conversion of toxins into harmless, water-soluble compounds. This interplay between nutrients and liver processes accentuates the criticality of a balanced diet in bolstering liver function and, by extension, ensuring overall health.

In a society quick to demonize cholesterol, a closer examination unveils a more nuanced reality. Cholesterol, far from being a mere villain, is essential for brain health and cellular function. The narrative that directly links high cholesterol to heart disease is oversimplified, overlooking the roles of inflammation and arterial damage. This chapter invites a reevaluation of cholesterol's reputation, advocating for a deeper understanding of its essential functions and the real contributors to heart disease. To cultivate liver health, a diet that minimizes refined carbohydrates and emphasizes fiber, protein, and healthy fats is paramount. The inclusion of liver-supportive herbs—dandelion, St. Mary's thistle (milk thistle), gentian, and ginger—offers additional fortification for liver function. This holistic dietary approach not only nurtures liver health but also paves the way for overall vitality and well-being, grounding us in a comprehensive understanding of nutrition's role in liver maintenance.

The prevalent reliance on cholesterol-lowering medications comes under scrutiny due to their associated risks, including cognitive and muscular side effects, and the potential for exacerbating diabetes and heart disease. This critical viewpoint underscores the necessity of prioritizing dietary and lifestyle modifications over pharmacological interventions. By embracing a holistic approach to cholesterol management, we can safeguard heart health more effectively and without the adverse effects associated with medication.

Heart Health

In the pursuit of heart health, our journey transcends traditional narratives, delving into a holistic understanding where lifestyle choices become the cornerstone of cardiovascular vitality. This comprehensive exploration navigates through the nuanced roles of cholesterol, dietary fats, the misunderstood implications of salt on blood pressure, and the natural alternatives for blood thinning, painting a picture of heart health that is both intricate and deeply interconnected. At the heart of cardiovascular wellness lies the undeniable truth that the heart, much more than a mere organ, is a dynamic muscle influenced profoundly by our daily choices. From the nourishment we provide through our diets to the energy we expend through physical activity, each decision weaves into the fabric of our vascular health. The heart, alongside the intricate network of blood and blood vessels, thrives on a balanced approach to living—highlighting the critical importance of fostering an environment conducive to heart health.

Venturing into the realm of cholesterol, long vilified in the discourse on heart disease, we encounter a narrative ripe for reevaluation. Cholesterol, a vital substance produced by the liver, is essential for myriad bodily functions, from cell repair to brain health. This narrative unfolds to reveal the distinction between HDL and LDL cholesterol—where HDL, the "good" cholesterol, acts as a guardian of cardiovascular health, and LDL, often misunderstood as purely harmful, plays a crucial role in the body's cellular architecture. This nuanced understanding challenges the oversimplified notion that cholesterol is the enemy, instead spotlighting the body's innate wisdom in managing cholesterol levels in harmony with our dietary intake. As we delve deeper, the conversation around dietary fats and heart health brings to light the complexity of our nutritional needs. The demonization of saturated fats, a staple in the diet of our ancestors, underscores a broader misunderstanding of fats' roles in our health. Embracing a diet that includes healthy fats, such as those found in coconut oil, offers a pathway to balanced nutrition, debunking myths and fostering a deeper appreciation for the varied functions fats perform in supporting our wellbeing.

The discourse on salt and its impact on blood pressure further exemplifies the need for a refined perspective on nutrition. Natural salts, rich in essential minerals, contrast sharply with their processed counterparts, offering a reminder of the importance of quality and source in our dietary choices. These natural salts, when consumed in moderation, contribute to a balanced diet, supporting heart health without the adverse effects often attributed to salt consumption. Lastly, the exploration of natural alternatives for blood thinning presents a compelling argument for the holistic management of cardiovascular health. Natural remedies such as water, cayenne pepper, garlic, and ginger emerge as powerful allies in promoting healthy circulation and combating inflammation. These alternatives, rooted in centuries of traditional wisdom, highlight the potential for natural substances to support heart health effectively, providing a complementary approach to conventional medications.

Brain Health

The journey to maintaining and enhancing brain health is an intricate dance of lifestyle choices, environmental factors, and spiritual well-being. Far from the inevitable decline many associate with aging, the brain is remarkably designed for longevity, equipped to become sharper and more intelligent over the years. This chapter delves into the foundations of brain health, from the pivotal role of the prefrontal cortex to the profound impact of forgiveness, nutrition, exercise, and spiritual harmony on our cognitive functions.

Central to our understanding of brain health is the recognition that the brain is inherently designed not to deteriorate but to thrive with age. The deterioration often observed in later years is not a natural consequence of aging but rather the result of lifestyle choices and environmental factors that can, fortunately, be modified. This perspective shifts the narrative from one of inevitable decline to a hopeful journey of continuous improvement and vitality. The prefrontal cortex stands as the brain's command center, playing a crucial role in reasoning, judgment, intellect, and willpower. It orchestrates decisions that shape our lives, from daily choices to our moral and ethical reasoning. Nurturing this part of the brain through stimulating activities and healthy lifestyle choices can significantly enhance its function, underscoring its importance in maintaining cognitive health.

Our daily habits profoundly influence brain health, with sleep, nutrition, hydration, exercise, and stress management acting as critical pillars. Adequate sleep, for instance, is essential for the brain's cleaning processes, clearing amyloid plaques linked to dementia and Alzheimer's. Similarly, nutrition rich in omega-3 fatty acids and hydration play pivotal roles in fueling the brain and supporting its overall health. Regular physical activity boosts blood circulation to the brain, ensuring a steady supply of oxygen and nutrients essential for cognitive function. The act of forgiveness emerges as a powerful tool for brain health, with the capacity to release the grip of negative emotions such as grief, anxiety, and unforgiveness that can physically damage the brain. Embracing forgiveness not only aids in mental health but also initiates a physiological healing process within the brain, rewiring and rejuvenating cognitive pathways.

Neuroplasticity, or the brain's ability to rewire itself, highlights the limitless potential for cognitive enhancement. Engaging in new learning activities stimulates the growth of dendrites, bolstering cognitive abilities and proving that our brains are capable of growth and adaptation at any age. Whether it's picking up a musical instrument, learning a new language, or engaging in mental exercises, each new challenge we introduce to our brain contributes to its vitality and longevity. A balanced diet, rich in essential nutrients like omega-3 fatty acids and whole salts, alongside adequate hydration, forms the foundation of brain nutrition. These elements are not merely fuel but are integral to the brain's energy production, functionality, and protection against cognitive decline. Incorporating spiritual practices and aligning one's life with biblical principles are highlighted as foundations for mental and spiritual well-being. Trust in God and adherence to the wisdom found in the Bible foster a sound mind and a peaceful life, contributing to overall brain health. This spiritual dimension adds a profound layer of support to the holistic approach to brain vitality, emphasizing the interconnectedness of mind, body, and spirit.

Book 2: Practical Implementation of Natural Healing

Daily Routines for Holistic Health

Integrating Barbara O'Neill's holistic health teachings into daily and weekly routines offers a practical roadmap for nurturing health and vitality amidst the hustle and bustle of modern life. This chapter aims to distill O'Neill's wisdom into actionable rituals that resonate with the rhythm of our daily lives, emphasizing the simplicity and power of natural healing.

Creating a Daily Routine

Morning Rituals

Hydration with a Mineral Boost: Beginning the day with hydration is transformed into a nourishing ritual by adding a small crystal of Celtic Sea salt to the first glass of water. This practice not only replenishes essential minerals but also enhances cellular hydration, setting a tone of mindfulness and self-care from the moment we wake. Imagine the difference in starting your day fully hydrated and mineral-replenished, ready to face the day's challenges with renewed energy.

Nourishing Breakfast: A breakfast rich in high-fiber foods, proteins from legumes, and healthy fats provides the foundation for sustained energy throughout the morning. A go-to meal could be a sprouted grain toast topped with mashed avocado and sprinkled with hemp seeds, offering a balance of nutrients that support both physical and cognitive functions. Such a meal not only satisfies hunger but also aligns with O'Neill's plant-based dietary principles, fueling the body with whole, unprocessed foods.

Midday Practices: Sustaining Energy and Focus

Mindful Eating: Lunch becomes an opportunity to practice mindful eating, consciously choosing ingredients that support holistic health. A salad packed with dark leafy greens, legumes such as black beans, and a homemade dressing rich in cold-pressed olive oil can provide a midday boost without the sluggishness often associated with heavier meals. This approach to lunch encourages not only nutritional balance but also a deeper connection with the food we consume.

Detoxification Support: Midday is also an ideal time to support the body's natural detoxification processes. Integrating a cup of herbal tea with liver-supporting herbs like dandelion or milk thistle into your routine can gently aid the liver, an organ pivotal to detoxification and overall vitality. Such small, intentional practices contribute significantly to the body's ability to heal and maintain balance.

Evening Wind-Down: Nurturing Rest and Recovery

Minimizing Exposure to Toxins: Dinner preparation offers a moment to apply O'Neill's guidance on reducing toxin exposure. Opting for simple, homemade meals with organic produce not only lessens the body's toxic burden but also ensures that the evening meal is a time of nourishment and relaxation. A simple yet flavorful dish could be baked sweet potatoes filled with a mix of sautéed kale, garlic, and chickpeas, drizzled with a tahini sauce, embodying the principles of whole, plant-based eating.

Addressing Specific Health Concerns: Evening routines can also focus on specific health concerns. For someone managing dry skin, incorporating a natural, herbal-infused moisturizer into their nighttime skincare routine can provide targeted healing. Similarly, including anti-inflammatory spices like turmeric in your dinner can support skin health from the inside out, illustrating how dietary choices can be tailored to address individual health needs.

Weekly Additions: Deepening the Practice

Embracing Seasonal Eating: O'Neill's emphasis on a plant-based diet rich in whole foods aligns beautifully with the practice of seasonal eating. Consuming fruits and vegetables that are in season not only ensures that you're getting the highest nutrient content but also supports local farming and reduces the environmental impact associated with long-distance food transportation. Dedicate one meal each week to exploring seasonal produce. This could involve visiting a local farmer's market or researching what's currently in season in your area. Prepare a meal centered around these finds, such as a roasted root vegetable dish in the winter or a fresh berry salad in the summer. This practice not only diversifies your nutrient intake but also introduces new flavors and dishes into your diet, making healthy eating an exciting and enjoyable adventure.

Legume Preparation: Setting aside time each week for the proper preparation of legumes can make these nutritious staples more accessible and digestible. A Sunday ritual of soaking, rinsing, and cooking a batch of beans or lentils ensures a ready supply of plant-based protein for the week ahead, embodying O'Neill's advice on enhancing nutrient absorption and minimizing digestive discomfort.

Creating a Weekly Herbal Ritual: Setting aside time each week to prepare and enjoy herbal infusions can significantly support digestive health, a cornerstone of O'Neill's approach to natural healing. Herbs like peppermint, ginger, and chamomile are not only soothing to the digestive tract but also offer a range of health benefits, from reducing inflammation to alleviating nausea. Select one day each week—perhaps a quiet Sunday evening or a mid-week break—to brew a large pot of herbal tea. Focus on herbs known for their digestive benefits. For example, a ginger tea can be made by simmering fresh ginger root in water for 15-20 minutes, while chamomile tea might be a gentle way to end the day, supporting not only digestion but also sleep. Store this infusion in the refrigerator and enjoy a cup each day, warming it slightly or drinking it at room temperature, to maintain a consistent aid for your digestive system throughout the week.

Practical Tips for Integrating Natural Remedies Into Everyday Life

In this chapter, we delve into practical advice for incorporating Barbara O'Neill's natural remedies into our lives, focusing not only on addressing specific health conditions but also on maintaining good health and preventing disease. By integrating these practices into our daily routines, we can harness the power of nature's remedies to support our body's inherent healing abilities.

Starting Your Day with Herbal Tonics

Begin each day with a herbal tonic to kickstart your digestion and boost your immune system. A simple yet effective tonic can be made from lemon, ginger, and a teaspoon of raw honey in warm water. This concoction aids in detoxification and provides anti-inflammatory benefits, making it an excellent preventive measure against colds and flu. Incorporate this tonic into your morning routine as you prepare breakfast, allowing the warm drink to stimulate your digestive system and awaken your senses, setting a positive tone for the day.

Integrating Herbal Teas for Hydration and Relaxation

Replace your afternoon coffee with a cup of herbal tea, such as peppermint or chamomile, which offer hydration and a calming effect on the mind and digestive system. In the midst of a busy workday, taking a moment to enjoy a cup of herbal tea can serve as a brief relaxation practice, reducing stress levels and supporting digestive health without the caffeine jitters.

Using Poultices and Compresses for Pain Relief

For acute conditions like joint pain or skin inflammation, prepare a ginger poultice or a castor oil compress. Apply these treatments in the evening, allowing the natural properties of the remedies to work as you rest. For example, after a day of intense physical activity or noticing the onset of joint discomfort, apply a ginger poultice to the affected area. This can alleviate inflammation and pain, enhancing recovery during sleep.

Daily Incorporation of Anti-inflammatory Foods

Make anti-inflammatory foods a staple in your diet. Incorporate turmeric into your cooking, add ground flaxseeds to your smoothies, and snack on nuts and seeds. These foods combat inflammation in the body, supporting overall health and preventing chronic conditions. Prepare a weekly meal plan that includes these anti-inflammatory ingredients in various meals, ensuring that every dish contributes to your body's well-being.

Enhancing Circulation with Cayenne Pepper

For those looking to improve circulation and cardiovascular health, adding a pinch of cayenne pepper to meals can provide circulatory benefits. Cayenne pepper can be especially beneficial during colder months when circulation might be compromised. Sprinkle cayenne pepper on your morning eggs or incorporate it into a warming soup. This not only adds flavor but also supports heart health and blood flow.

Charcoal Poultices for Emergency Detoxification

Keep activated charcoal on hand for emergencies involving bites, stings, or sudden allergic reactions. Creating a charcoal poultice can quickly absorb toxins and reduce swelling. f you enjoy hiking or outdoor activities, having activated charcoal in your first aid kit can provide a natural and effective remedy for unexpected insect bites or contact with irritants.

Regular Hydrotherapy for Muscle Relaxation

Dedicate one evening a week to a relaxing Epsom salt bath. This practice can soothe sore muscles, reduce stress, and prepare your body for restorative sleep. Choose a day that tends to be your most stressful or physically demanding, and let this hydrotherapy session be a healing closure, allowing you to unwind and recharge.

By embedding these natural remedies and practices into our daily and weekly routines, we cultivate a lifestyle centered around prevention and holistic well-being. The key is consistency and intentionality, allowing the cumulative effect of these practices to support our health journey. Whether it's starting the day with a nourishing tonic, finding moments of calm with herbal teas, or preparing for rest with hydrotherapy, each step is a building block towards achieving optimal health, guided by the wisdom of Barbara O'Neill's natural healing teachings.

Nurturing Personal Hygiene, Sleep, and Stress Management Naturally

In the realm of holistic health, personal hygiene, sleep quality, and effective stress management form the pillars of a balanced lifestyle. Drawing from the wealth of natural remedies and practices, this chapter introduces innovative and perhaps less familiar strategies. By adopting these natural means, we can enhance our well-being, ensuring that our daily routines support a life of vitality and tranquility

Personal Hygiene with Natural Antiseptics

Tea Tree Oil: Renowned for its antimicrobial properties, tea tree oil serves as an excellent natural antiseptic for skin care and wound healing. Incorporate tea tree oil into your daily hygiene routine by adding a few drops to your bathwater or mixing it with a carrier oil for a natural disinfectant for cuts and scrapes.

Neem: A powerhouse in natural health, neem possesses antibacterial and antifungal qualities, making it ideal for oral hygiene. Consider adding neem oil to your homemade toothpaste or seeking out neem-based dental care products to reduce plaque and prevent gingivitis, naturally promoting oral health.

Real-life Application: For those prone to skin irritations or looking to enhance their oral health regimen, integrating tea tree oil and neem into your personal care routine can offer effective, chemical-free alternatives to conventional antiseptics.

Enhancing Sleep Quality with Aromatic Herbs

Lavender and Chamomile: While these herbs are well-known for their calming effects, their application extends beyond teas. Create a bedtime ritual by using lavender and chamomile essential oils in a diffuser to promote relaxation and enhance sleep quality. The soothing aroma eases the mind into a state conducive to restful sleep.

Hops: Less commonly recognized for its sedative properties, hops can be used to improve sleep. Filling a small sachet with dried hops and placing it under your pillow can help deepen sleep naturally, offering an alternative for those seeking novel remedies for insomnia.

For anyone struggling with sleep disturbances, crafting a nightly routine that incorporates these aromatic herbs can transform your bedroom into a sanctuary for rest, aiding in the natural transition to sleep.

Stress Management with Adaptogens and Water Therapy

Rhodiola and Holy Basil: As adaptogens, rhodiola and holy basil support the body's natural response to stress and fatigue. Incorporating these herbs into your diet through supplements or herbal teas can enhance resilience to stress, improving mental clarity and energy levels.

Water Therapy: Embracing practices like cold showers or alternating between hot and cold water can invigorate the body and reduce stress. This form of hydrotherapy stimulates circulation and enhances mental alertness, providing a refreshing start to the day or a revitalizing break when stress levels rise.

In the face of a stressful period at work or during times of high emotional strain, integrating adaptogens like rhodiola and holy basil into your daily regimen, combined with invigorating water therapy practices, can offer a holistic approach to managing stress, keeping you balanced and focused.

Cultivating a Healthy Gut with Fermented Foods

Kefir and Sauerkraut: Beyond the well-trodden path of probiotic supplements lies the rich terrain of fermented foods, such as kefir and sauerkraut, which naturally enhance gut health. These fermented wonders are not only teeming with probiotics but also introduce a diversity of beneficial bacteria to the digestive system, supporting digestion and bolstering the immune system. Integrating kefir into your morning smoothie or adding a serving of sauerkraut to your daily meals can significantly improve gut flora balance. For those experiencing digestive discomfort or seeking to maintain optimal gut health, the inclusion of kefir and sauerkraut in your diet offers a delicious and natural way to nurture your digestive system. Imagine the transformation in your digestive health as you make these fermented foods a staple in your kitchen, enjoying the tangy flavors while nourishing your gut microbiome.

Calendula and Rosehip Oil: Venturing into the realm of natural skincare, the healing properties of calendula and the regenerative benefits of rosehip oil present a luxurious yet simple approach to maintaining radiant skin. Calendula, with its soothing properties, is perfect for calming irritated skin, while rosehip oil, rich in vitamins and antioxidants, promotes skin regeneration and reduces scars and fine lines. Creating a nightly skincare ritual that includes these herbal oils can enhance skin health, providing a natural glow without the need for chemical-laden products. Imagine ending your day by gently massaging a blend of calendula and rosehip oil into your skin, not only as an act of self-care but also as a way to naturally support skin healing and rejuvenation. This practice not only benefits the skin but also offers a moment of relaxation and connection with nature's healing touch.

Herbal Remedies and Their Applications

In the expansive realm of nature's pharmacy, herbs emerge as quintessential allies in the quest for health and vitality. This section ventures deep into the herbal lore, presenting an all-encompassing tutorial on embracing these natural wonders. Tracing a lineage from age-old traditions to contemporary holistic methodologies, herbs have consistently been celebrated for their therapeutic virtues. Channeling insights parallel to Barbara O'Neill's integrative perspective, this narrative embarks on a journey to leverage herbal potency for enhancing our day-to-day wellness.

Comprehensive Guide to Herbs for Health and Wellness

Herbs are endowed with an impressive spectrum of healing attributes, each providing distinct advantages for our health. For example, antimicrobial herbs such as garlic and oregano combat infections by thwarting the proliferation of bacteria and viruses. Anti-inflammatory herbs, like turmeric and ginger, alleviate inflammation, easing ailments such as arthritis and digestive woes. Adaptogens, such as ashwagandha and holy basil, fortify the body's stress response, stabilizing bodily processes.

Crafting Herbal Remedies

The craft of concocting herbal solutions entails pinpointing the optimal herb(s) for a given health issue or objective. These remedies can manifest in several forms, including teas, tinctures, capsules, poultices, and oils, each offering varied benefits in terms of strength, absorption, and convenience.

Teas: Perfect for mild, routine support, herbal teas involve infusing dried herbs in boiling water. Peppermint tea, for instance, can alleviate digestive problems, while chamomile tea aids in relaxation and sleep.

Tinctures: Potent herbal extracts created by immersing herbs in alcohol or vinegar to draw out their powerful elements. Administered in minor doses, tinctures serve as robust treatments for various conditions, from bolstering immunity to easing stress.

Essential Oils, the essence of plant's vigor, are garnered through steam distillation or cold pressing, spotlighting their dynamic aromatic essences. Lavender, known for its tranquility, and eucalyptus, celebrated for respiratory wellness, stand as pillars in aromatherapy, air diffusion, or when melded with carrier oils for skin application. Embedding essential oils into daily rituals, such as sprinkling a few droplets into a bath or utilizing them in a nocturnal diffuser, markedly amplifies well-being and caters to specific health requisites.

Decoctions, a technique of simmering robust plant parts like roots, bark, and seeds, unveil their core nutrients over prolonged heat exposure. This approach excels with sturdy herbs demanding intense extraction for their prized compounds. A burdock root decoction acts as a formidable blood cleanser, whereas cinnamon bark decoction can aid in blood sugar stabilization. Weaving decoctions into your health regimen, particularly in the chill of winter, bestows warming and fortifying advantages.

Mother Tinctures, dense herbal extracts, emerge from marinating fresh or dried herbs in an alcohol-water amalgam. As the cornerstone for homeopathic dilutions, they encapsulate the herb's remedial essence. A milk thistle mother tincture supports liver vitality, presenting a direct and robust botanical cure. Incorporating mother tinctures into daily wellness strategies offers an efficient method to exploit herbal therapeutic benefits.

Poultices and Oils: For external use, poultices made of fresh or dried herbs applied to the skin can mitigate local inflammation and discomfort. Herbal oils, enriched with herbs like calendula or lavender, moisturize the skin and facilitate healing.

Other Herbal Preparations

Herbal Syrups merge decoctions or tinctures with honey or sugar, creating a delightful herbal intake mode, particularly enticing for children or those who disdain raw herb flavors. Elderberry syrup, a favored pick for immune enhancement during flu season, exemplifies this.

Herbal Baths immerse herbs or their extracts in bathwater, crafting a serene and healing soak. A chamomile and lavender bath preludes sleep with calm, whereas rosemary and peppermint invigorate and bolster circulation.

Herbal Compresses, achieved by drenching a cloth in an herbal infusion or decoction and applying it locally, address specific areas in need. An arnica-infused compress excellently mitigates bruising and swelling, providing focused comfort.

Personalizing Herbal Applications

Tailoring herbal practices to your specific requirements and inclinations is crucial. Capsules or tinctures might suit those with hectic schedules, offering an easy method to harness herbal benefits. For skin conditions, topical applications such as poultices or oils may be more suitable. Begin with minimal doses to monitor your body's reaction, and seek advice from a healthcare provider, especially if you are pregnant, breastfeeding, or on medications.

Stress and Anxiety: Adaptogenic herbs like ashwagandha, in tincture or capsule form, can diminish stress and enhance adaptability. A nightly routine of sipping chamomile or lemon balm tea can foster relaxation and improved sleep.

Digestive Health: Daily consumption of ginger or peppermint tea can support digestion and alleviate indigestion and nausea symptoms. For immediate issues, a fennel seed tincture offers rapid relief from gas and bloating.

Skin Care: For those exploring natural skin remedies, applying calendula-infused oil can relieve dry, irritated skin, whereas diluted tea tree oil can tackle acne and inflammation.

Immune Support: Herbs like echinacea and elderberry are formidable in augmenting the immune system. Regular intake of echinacea tea or elderberry syrup during cold and flu season can bolster your body's defenses.

Incorporating herbal remedies into our routines allows us to connect with the enduring knowledge of natural healing, empowering us to care for our health in a holistic manner. This exploration into the realm of herbal health and wellness invites you to delve into the vast world of herbal medicine, where each plant offers a pathway to enhanced health, vitality, and harmony with the natural world.

Customizing herbal treatments for individual needs

Acknowledging each person's distinctiveness is fundamental. Tailoring herbal remedies to align with individual health requisites and inclinations is a key pillar of efficacious natural therapy. This discourse ventures into the craft and science of customizing herbal treatments, ensuring they cater to our body's unique needs, lifestyle, and wellness ambitions. By embracing a bespoke approach to herbal medicine, we amplify the curative potential of herbs, bolstering our well-being and propelling us towards peak health.

The initiation of bespoke herbal strategies requires a comprehensive analysis of one's health status. This encompasses understanding prevailing health conditions, medical background, allergies, and distinct wellness objectives. For instance, an individual grappling with persistent inflammation may find solace in anti-inflammatory herbs such as turmeric or ginger, while someone facing stress and anxiety might derive benefits from adaptogenic herbs like ashwagandha or rhodiola. Adapting herbal solutions also means reflecting on one's lifestyle and personal tastes. For those ensnared in a hectic life, convenience may be paramount, tilting the balance towards tinctures or capsules rather than teas or decoctions demanding time to prepare. Taste predilections might also steer the choice of herbs or their consumption form, ensuring the remedy is not only potent but palatable.

Grasping the synergistic potential of herb pairings can markedly boost the effectiveness of herbal concoctions. Merging herbs with complementary healing attributes can forge potent blends tackling various facets of a health issue. For instance, unifying echinacea, celebrated for its immune-enhancing prowess, with elderberry, known for its antiviral advantages, can forge a formidable concoction for cold and flu prevention and mitigation. Identifying the correct dosage and treatment duration is pivotal in customization. Variables like age, weight, and condition severity influence the herb quantity and usage span. Incremental adjustments and response monitoring are vital to pinpoint the ideal dosage, maximizing benefits while dodging undesirable effects.

Adhering to customization principles in herbal medicine allows for the crafting of personalized healing plans that honor our unique health profiles and preferences. This tailored methodology not only elevates herbal remedy efficacy but also engages individuals actively in their health and healing odyssey, deepening the bond with nature and its restorative gifts.

The Role of Physical Activity and Mindfulness

Exercises and Activities Recommended

The synergy of physical exertion and mindfulness crafts a dynamic narrative that uplifts every facet of our existence. This harmonious blend of kinetic energy and mental acuity forms the essence of a lifestyle dedicated to fostering vitality, resilience, and serenity. Drawing from holistic health principles, this discourse navigates the integration of physical activities, with a special emphasis on the revitalizing art of rebounding, alongside mindfulness strategies, into a unified regimen promoting enduring health and vitality across the lifespan.

Embarking on this holistic health voyage is a lifelong pledge that defies the boundaries of age. Inspirational narratives of senior athletes exemplify that achieving and maintaining a vigorous, healthy body in our later years is not merely a possibility but a tangible goal for those committed to regular physical engagement. These stories shine as guiding lights, marking the trail for our personal health endeavors and prompting us to ponder our current preparations for achieving the health and vigor we desire in our later days. Highlighting the importance of physical readiness for our later years underscores that our present-day decisions are the bedrock of our future life quality. Engaging in consistent exercise transcends being a mere routine; it's a forward-looking investment in our future selves, ensuring we sustain our activity, autonomy, and zest as we age. In this preventative health strategy, High-Intensity Interval Training (HIIT) stands out for its efficacy. Defined by swift, intense activity spurts followed by rest intervals, HIIT epitomizes the efficiency our contemporary life demands. Requiring as brief as 15 minutes daily, HIIT exemplifies that exercise's quality can surpass quantity. Its advantages extend beyond saving time, enhancing circulation, lung function, and heart robustness—crucial factors in curtailing aging-related physical decline.

Exploring the cellular impact, exercises like HIIT profoundly influence our bodies. They enhance metabolic functions such as glycolysis and the Krebs cycle, optimizing lactic acid conversion back to pyruvate during rest, thus underlining exercise's supportive role in muscle and overall metabolic health. Additionally, the surge of Human Growth

Hormone (HGH) during physical activity is instrumental in health maintenance, facilitating fat metabolism, protein synthesis, and circulation enhancement, collectively decelerating the aging trajectory. Rebounding, or mini-trampoline bouncing, occupies a unique niche in holistic health-supportive exercises. Lauded for its extensive benefits, rebounding transcends exercise; it's a kinetic celebration that activates the lymphatic system, bolsters balance, and fortifies the body comprehensively. Rebounding's allure stems from its simplicity and the joy embedded in the exercise routine, fostering long-term adherence and enjoyment.

Blending mindfulness with physical activity transcends conventional exercise, morphing it into a holistic ritual that feeds the mind, soul, and body. Mindfulness, the practice of inhabiting the moment fully, transforms physical exertion into an all-encompassing ritual that deepens self-connection and augments overall well-being. Whether it's through concentrated breathing in a HIIT workout, the rhythmic motion on a mini-trampoline, or the intentional strides of a mindful stroll, this amalgamation of mindfulness with movement invites a profound self-relation, enriching our total health. Weaving these practices into daily life shouldn't be daunting. It involves seizing daily moments for mindful motion, be it a morning HIIT routine to invigorate the day's onset, a noon rebounding session to refresh mind and body, or an evening contemplative walk to decompress and contemplate. Approaching each activity with purpose and mindfulness crafts a holistic health regimen that nurtures not only physical but also emotional and mental well-being.

Mindfulness and Meditation Practices for Mental Health

Mindfulness, the art of being fully present and engaged in the moment without judgment, invites us to experience life more deeply and fully. It teaches us to observe our thoughts, feelings, and sensations as they are, providing a foundation of self-awareness and compassion. Meditation, a practice deeply intertwined with mindfulness, offers a structured approach to cultivating this awareness, through focused attention or open monitoring of our inner experiences. Together, these practices serve as a beacon, guiding us toward tranquility in the midst of life's storms. The application of mindfulness and meditation in daily life acts as a gentle yet powerful antidote to stress, anxiety, and depression. By learning to anchor ourselves in the present moment, we can navigate life's challenges with greater ease and perspective. These practices encourage a shift from reactive patterns to responsive presence, allowing us to meet each moment with a sense of clarity and choice.

Integrating mindfulness into daily routines can begin with simple, intentional actions. It might be the mindful savoring of a morning cup of tea, where we fully immerse ourselves in the experience—the warmth of the cup, the aroma of the tea, the taste on our lips. This deliberate attention to the present moment can then extend to other activities, transforming mundane tasks into opportunities for presence and mindfulness. Creating space for regular meditation practice is akin to planting a garden of tranquility in our minds. Starting with just a few minutes each day, we can explore various forms of meditation, such as breath awareness, guided imagery, or loving-kindness meditation, to find what resonates with our unique mental landscape. This dedicated time becomes a sanctuary, a place to return to for grounding and centering amidst the day's demands. Mindfulness can also be woven into physical activities, blurring the lines between movement and meditation. Practices like yoga, tai chi, or even mindful walking integrate the awareness of breath and movement, fostering a meditative state that nurtures both body and mind. Engaging in these activities not only supports physical health but also deepens the mindfulness practice, illustrating the interconnectedness of our physical and mental well-being.

As we deepen our mindfulness and meditation practices, we may notice a ripple effect—improvements in areas of life beyond immediate mental health. Relationships can become more authentic and compassionate, work may feel more purposeful and less stressful, and everyday challenges are met with increased resilience and equanimity. Encountering distractions and resistance is a natural part of cultivating mindfulness and meditation practices. Approaching these challenges with self-compassion and curiosity rather than criticism allows us to learn from our experiences and deepen our practice. It's in these moments of struggle that the true transformative potential of mindfulness and meditation is often realized.

Balancing Physical Activity With Rest and Recovery

In the holistic approach to health and wellness, the equilibrium between physical activity and rest encapsulates a fundamental principle: true strength and vitality are nurtured not just through exertion but equally through periods of recovery and stillness. This chapter delves into the intricate dance of balancing vigorous physical activity with the essential, rejuvenating phases of rest and recovery, a rhythm that mirrors the natural cycles of action and repose inherent in life itself.

At the heart of this balance is the understanding that physical activity, while vital for maintaining health, places demands on the body that must be counterbalanced by adequate rest. Exercise stimulates muscle growth, enhances cardiovascular health, and boosts mental well-being, among numerous other benefits. Yet, it is in the moments of rest that the body undertakes the critical processes of repair, strengthening, and adaptation. Recognizing this synergy is crucial; *have you ever considered how your rest days are as important as your workout sessions?*

Active recovery, an approach that combines gentle movement with rest days, serves as a bridge between intense physical exertion and complete rest. Activities like light walking, yoga, or stretching maintain the flow of circulation, aiding the body in its natural repair processes without imposing undue stress. This method not only accelerates recovery but also maintains a connection to the joy and habit of movement, preventing the inertia that can accompany complete rest. A key to balancing activity with rest is attuning to the body's signals. Symptoms like prolonged fatigue, decreased performance, or irritability can be indicators of inadequate recovery. Cultivating an awareness of these signs enables us to adjust our routines, perhaps incorporating more rest or modifying the intensity of our workouts. This attentiveness to the body's needs fosters a deeper harmony within our physical and mental realms.

Integrating structured rest days into your exercise routine is not a pause in progress but a vital component of it. Planning rest days allows the body to recuperate and rebuild, preparing for the next phase of activity with renewed strength and vitality. Moreover, these days offer an opportunity to engage in mindfulness or meditative practices, enhancing the recovery process by addressing the mental and emotional aspects of well-being. Balancing physical activity with rest also involves mindful nourishment. Consuming a diet rich in whole foods, proteins, healthy fats, and carbohydrates supports the body's repair processes. Hydration, too, plays a critical role in recovery, replenishing fluids lost during exercise and aiding in cellular repair.

Ultimately, balancing physical activity with rest and recovery embodies a holistic view of health, recognizing that our well-being is nurtured not by relentless exertion but through a respectful partnership between action and stillness. This perspective invites us to honor our body's rhythms, to find joy in both movement and rest, and to appreciate the profound wisdom in nature's cycles of activity and recovery.

Book 3: Advanced Natural Healing Techniques

Advanced Detoxification and Cleansing Methods

Our bodies are exposed to an array of toxins daily, from environmental pollutants and processed foods to stress and sedentary lifestyles. While the body possesses innate detoxification systems, the overload of these toxins can impede its ability to cleanse effectively. Advanced detoxification practices are designed to support and amplify the body's natural detox mechanisms, targeting deeper layers of toxin accumulation and facilitating their elimination. Advanced detoxification is grounded in a holistic understanding of the body's systems, emphasizing the need to cleanse not just the physical body but also the mental and emotional layers of our being. This comprehensive approach ensures that detoxification is not merely a physical process but a transformative experience that nurtures the whole person.

Key Advanced Detoxification Practices

Fasting and Juice Cleanses: Going beyond intermittent fasting, extended fasting or juice cleanses offer a profound way to rest the digestive system and mobilize deep-seated toxins. These practices should be approached with caution and ideally under the guidance of a healthcare professional to ensure they are conducted safely and effectively.

Herbal Detoxification Protocols: Certain herbs, known for their potent cleansing properties, can be incorporated into a detox regimen to support liver function, kidney health, and lymphatic drainage. Herbs such as milk thistle, dandelion root, and burdock can be used in specific formulations to enhance detoxification.

Colon Cleansing: Techniques such as colon hydrotherapy or the use of herbal colon cleansers aim to remove waste material and toxins from the colon. This practice can be an integral part of an advanced detoxification protocol, improving gut health and enhancing the body's ability to eliminate toxins.

Sauna Therapy and Sweat Lodges: Utilizing heat to induce sweating, sauna therapy, and sweat lodges are traditional practices that support toxin elimination through the skin. These methods, combined with hydration and mineral replenishment, can significantly aid the detoxification process.

Chelation Therapy: For heavy metal detoxification, chelation therapy involves the administration of chelating agents that bind to heavy metals in the body, facilitating their excretion. This advanced detox method should only be undertaken with medical supervision due to its potent effects and potential risks.

Recognizing the interconnectedness of the physical, mental, and emotional realms, advanced detoxification also encompasses practices that address emotional and psychological toxins. Mindfulness meditation, breathwork, and journaling can be powerful tools for releasing emotional baggage, reducing stress, and supporting mental clarity during the detox process. Embarking on advanced detoxification requires careful consideration of one's health status, goals, and any potential risks. Consulting with healthcare professionals experienced in detoxification is crucial to tailoring these practices to individual needs and ensuring they are conducted safely. Listening to the body and honoring its signals throughout the detox process is also vital, allowing for adjustments as needed to support health and well-being.

In-Depth Guidance On Advanced Detox Methods

Advanced detoxification methods offer profound ways to cleanse the body, enhance vitality, and support overall wellness. By delving into specific techniques and providing actionable, real-life examples, this section aims to guide individuals on how to effectively incorporate these practices into their health regimen.

Herbal Detoxification Protocols

Creating a daily detox tea blend can be a practical way to incorporate detoxifying herbs into your routine. For example, a morning tea made from dandelion root, milk thistle, and burdock offers a powerful combination to support liver function and promote bile flow, essential for breaking down fats and eliminating toxins. Dandelion root acts as a diuretic, supporting kidney health, while milk thistle is renowned for its liver-protective effects, and burdock root aids in lymphatic drainage and blood purification. Start your day with a warm cup of this herbal detox tea. Steep one teaspoon each of dried dandelion root, milk thistle seeds, and burdock root in hot water for about 10-15 minutes. Strain and enjoy this cleansing beverage first thing in the morning to kickstart your body's natural detoxification processes.

Colon Cleansing

Integrating a gentle, herbal colon cleanse into your detox plan can effectively remove waste material and support gut health. A simple and natural approach involves using psyllium husk, a fiber that acts as a natural laxative, and aloe vera, which soothes and heals the intestinal lining. For one week, mix a tablespoon of psyllium husk in water and drink it each night before bed, followed by a small glass of aloe vera juice. Ensure to increase your water intake during this period to facilitate the cleansing process. This regimen can help clear the colon, promoting effective toxin elimination and improving digestive function.

Sauna Therapy and Sweat Lodges

Incorporating sauna sessions into your weekly routine can significantly enhance toxin elimination through the skin. For those without access to a traditional sauna, portable infrared saunas offer a convenient at-home alternative, delivering deep tissue warmth and promoting detoxifying sweat. Schedule 2-3 sauna sessions per week, gradually increasing the duration from 15 to 30 minutes per session. Ensure to hydrate well before and after, drinking electrolyte-rich fluids or water with a pinch of Himalayan salt to replenish minerals lost through sweating. Following each session, take a cool shower to remove toxins from the skin's surface and close the pores, enhancing the cleansing effect.

Precautions and How to Tailor Detoxification

Embarking on a detoxification journey necessitates a deep understanding of one's own body and health status, emphasizing the importance of a personalized approach to ensure safety and effectiveness. The process of detoxification, while beneficial, carries with it the responsibility to proceed with caution, particularly when navigating the vast landscape of detox methods available. This narrative seeks to guide individuals through tailoring detox practices to their unique health needs, ensuring that each step taken contributes positively to their overall well-being.

Before delving into any detox regimen, it's imperative to conduct a thorough assessment of one's health. This holistic overview, considering factors such as existing health conditions, medications, and lifestyle, lays the groundwork for selecting detox practices that harmonize with the individual's body. Consulting with healthcare professionals experienced in detoxification offers a foundational step, providing insights and oversight that tailor the detox process to align with personal health goals and conditions. This collaboration ensures that chosen methods are not only safe but optimized for efficacy. Starting slowly allows the body to adjust to the changes. Beginning with less intensive practices, such as incorporating detoxifying foods and engaging in gentle sauna sessions, sets a sustainable pace. Listening to the body's responses during this process is crucial; it communicates when adjustments are needed or when a practice may be too intense. Recognizing and respecting these signals is key to a successful detoxification experience.

Detoxification can, at times, elicit a range of responses, from mild fatigue to more pronounced symptoms such as headaches or digestive changes. These reactions, often signs of the body's adjustment to the detox process, require careful attention. Severe or persistent symptoms signal the need to reevaluate the intensity of the detox, underscoring the importance of a tailored approach that respects the body's limits. Personalizing detox methods involves selecting practices that resonate with the individual's specific health profile. For someone with a sensitive digestive system, gentle herbal teas and dietary modifications may provide a supportive detox experience without the harshness of more aggressive methods. In contrast, individuals with certain health conditions should approach practices like sauna therapy with caution, opting for milder forms of sweating and detoxification that do not compromise their health.

Also, nutritional support plays a pivotal role in the detoxification process, providing the body with the essential nutrients needed to support and enhance detox organs. Tailoring one's diet to include foods that bolster detoxification, coupled with supplements to replenish lost nutrients, under the guidance of a healthcare professional, ensures that the body receives comprehensive support throughout the detox process. Incorporating rest and mental detox into the regimen acknowledges the interconnectedness of physical and mental well-being. Allowing time for recovery, integrating mindfulness practices, and ensuring adequate sleep complement the physical aspects of detox, offering a holistic approach that nurtures both body and mind. Viewing detoxification as part of a broader, long-term wellness strategy emphasizes the importance of integrating healthy lifestyle practices beyond the detox period. This perspective encourages a sustained commitment to well-being, where regular physical activity, a balanced diet, and stress management continue to support the body's natural healing processes.

Monitoring Progress and Adjusting Practices

Navigating the path of detoxification is akin to embarking on a personal journey of discovery and renewal, where monitoring progress and making adjustments are integral to achieving optimal health outcomes. This dynamic process requires attentiveness and flexibility, as the body's responses to detox practices can offer valuable insights into what is working well and what might need refinement.

- **The Importance of Regular Check-Ins:** Establishing regular check-ins with oneself is crucial for monitoring the effects of detoxification practices. These moments of reflection can involve assessing physical symptoms, energy levels, emotional well-being, and overall sense of vitality. Keeping a journal can be particularly effective, offering a tangible record of observations and changes over time. This practice not only aids in recognizing patterns and shifts in well-being but also fosters a deeper connection to one's health journey.

- **Listening to the Body's Signals:** The body communicates in nuanced ways, signaling when it is thriving and when it is under strain. Symptoms such as increased energy, improved digestion, and clearer skin can indicate positive progress in the detox process. Conversely, signs of fatigue, irritability, or discomfort may suggest that certain practices are too intense or not aligned with the body's current needs. Attuning to these signals is a vital skill, enabling individuals to respond with adjustments that support healing and balance.

- **The Role of Professional Guidance:** Consulting with healthcare professionals throughout the detox journey offers an additional layer of insight and support. These experts can provide objective assessments of progress, suggest modifications, and address any concerns that arise. Their guidance is particularly valuable for interpreting the body's signals accurately and making informed decisions about adjusting detox practices. Regular consultations ensure that the detoxification process remains safe, effective, and aligned with individual health goals.

- **Adapting Practices for Sustained Well-being:** Adjusting detox practices is not a sign of setback but rather a reflection of the body's evolving needs and the deepening understanding of one's health. This might involve modifying the intensity or duration of certain practices, introducing new detox methods, or even taking breaks to allow the body to rest. Flexibility and responsiveness to change are key, allowing the detox process to be a nurturing, rather than rigid, experience.

- **Integrating New Habits for Long-term Health:** As individuals progress through their detox journey, certain practices may resonate deeply, offering benefits that extend beyond the detoxification period. Integrating these practices into daily life can contribute to long-term health and vitality. For example, if regular sauna sessions prove beneficial, making them a consistent part of one's wellness routine can continue to support toxin elimination and relaxation. Similarly, dietary changes adopted during detox, such as increased consumption of whole foods and hydration, can lay the foundation for lasting dietary habits that promote health and prevent disease.

- **Celebrating Progress and Reevaluating Goals:** Monitoring progress also involves recognizing and celebrating milestones, however small they may seem. Acknowledging the steps taken towards improved health can be incredibly motivating, reinforcing the value of the detoxification journey. Additionally, as individuals achieve certain health objectives, it may be time to reevaluate goals, setting new targets that reflect their current health status and aspirations.

Specialized Natural Therapies

Exploration of Specialized Therapies

Beginning a journey of holistic health invites the exploration of specialized therapies that complement traditional wellness practices. Among these, hydrotherapy, aromatherapy, and reflexology stand out for their unique abilities to heal and rejuvenate your body and mind. This chapter delves into the essence of these therapies, uncovering their principles, benefits, and practical applications, offering a gateway to enhanced well-being through nature's own remedies.

- **Hydrotherapy:** The therapeutic use of water in its various forms and temperatures, harnesses water's natural properties to heal, soothe, and revitalize. This ancient practice, which spans from hot springs baths to cold compresses, operates on the principle that water can stimulate the body's self-healing mechanisms. Incorporating hydrotherapy into your wellness routine can be as simple as alternating between hot and cold showers to stimulate circulation and immune response. For deeper therapeutic effects, soaking in an Epsom salt bath can relieve muscle tension and promote relaxation, while targeted cold therapy, such as ice packs on inflamed areas, can reduce swelling and pain. These practices, easily integrated into daily life, offer a testament to water's profound healing capabilities.

- **Aromatherapy:** This therapy utilizes the aromatic compounds found in plants, distilled into essential oils, to influence mood, health, and cognitive function. This therapy is grounded in the understanding that the inhalation and topical application of these oils can have therapeutic effects on the body and mind, tapping into the ancient wisdom of plant medicine. To harness the benefits of aromatherapy, consider diffusing lavender oil in your bedroom to promote restful sleep or peppermint oil in your workspace to enhance concentration and energy. For physical ailments, applying diluted eucalyptus oil to the chest can alleviate respiratory congestion, while a blend of chamomile and frankincense oils can soothe skin irritations. The versatility of essential oils allows for personalized blends that cater to individual needs and preferences, making aromatherapy a highly adaptable and potent tool in holistic health.

- **Reflexology:** A practice that applies pressure to specific points on the feet, hands, and ears, is based on the premise that these points correspond to different organs and systems within the body. By stimulating these reflex points, reflexology aims to promote balance, alleviate pain, and support overall health. Integrating reflexology into your wellness regime can begin with self-applied pressure to areas corresponding to tension or discomfort. For instance, massaging the reflex points related to the head and neck on your feet can offer relief from headaches. Seeking out a professional reflexologist can further enhance the therapeutic benefits, providing a tailored approach to addressing specific health concerns through targeted reflexology sessions.

The exploration of hydrotherapy, aromatherapy, and reflexology reveals a world of specialized therapies that complement and enhance traditional health practices. Each therapy offers unique pathways to healing, grounded in the understanding that our connection to natural elements—water, plants, and the body's own reflex points—can unlock profound health benefits.

How These Therapies Can Be Integrated Into a Holistic Healing Plan

Integrating specialized therapies into a holistic healing plan offers a multi-faceted approach to wellness, addressing not just the physical aspects of health but also the emotional and mental dimensions. This integration fosters a comprehensive healing environment, where each therapy complements the others, creating a synergy that amplifies overall well-being. This chapter explores how to weave these specialized therapies into a cohesive holistic healing plan, offering practical strategies for achieving a balanced and harmonious state of health.

Creating a Foundation with Hydrotherapy

With its versatile applications, Hydrotherapy serves as a foundational element in a holistic healing plan. Its ability to manipulate circulation through temperature changes makes it an excellent starting point for addressing a variety of health concerns, from stress and anxiety to chronic pain and inflammation. Begin by identifying specific health goals, such as reducing muscle tension or improving sleep quality. Incorporate daily or weekly hydrotherapy practices aligned with these goals. For instance, if reducing stress is a priority, establish a routine of nightly warm baths infused with calming essential oils like lavender. For those seeking relief from muscle soreness or joint pain, alternating hot and cold showers may offer significant benefits, stimulating blood flow and reducing inflammation.

Enhancing Emotional and Mental Well-being with Aromatherapy

Aromatherapy's power to influence mood and cognitive function makes it an invaluable component of a holistic healing plan, particularly for managing stress, anxiety, and mood fluctuations.Integrate aromatherapy into daily routines to create an atmosphere that supports emotional and mental well-being. Use diffusers with uplifting citrus oils in the morning to set a positive tone for the day, and switch to soothing scents like chamomile or sandalwood in the evening to promote relaxation. For targeted emotional support, carry a small bottle of a comforting essential oil blend to inhale during moments of stress or fatigue.

Balancing the Plan with Reflexology

Reflexology adds a layer of therapeutic touch to the holistic healing plan, offering a hands-on method for stimulating the body's healing processes and enhancing overall vitality. Map out a weekly reflexology routine, focusing on areas that correspond to specific health concerns identified in your holistic plan. For self-applied reflexology, dedicate a few minutes each day to massaging reflex points on the hands or feet that relate to areas of tension or imbalance. Incorporating professional reflexology sessions monthly can provide deeper therapeutic benefits, with tailored treatments that support your specific wellness goals.

Harmonizing Therapies for Optimal Health

The true art of integrating specialized therapies into a holistic healing plan lies in creating a harmonious balance that respects the body's natural rhythms and healing capacity. This involves not only scheduling each therapy strategically throughout the week but also tuning into the body's responses, adjusting practices as needed to align with changing health needs and goals. This integrated strategy not only addresses specific health concerns but also promotes a deeper sense of well-being, empowering individuals to live more balanced, healthy, and harmonious lives. Keep in mind to maintain a reflective practice, noting changes in your physical, emotional, and mental well-being. This ongoing assessment allows for the holistic plan to evolve, incorporating more or less of each therapy as your health journey progresses. The flexibility to adapt and tailor the healing plan is key to achieving lasting wellness.

Practical Advice For Beginners

Embarking on a journey of holistic healing can seem daunting to beginners, especially when considering the integration of specialized therapies like hydrotherapy, aromatherapy, and reflexology into daily life. This chapter aims to demystify these practices, offering practical advice and a step-by-step plan to seamlessly incorporate these natural therapies into your wellness routine, fostering a balanced and harmonious approach to health.

- **Starting Small with Hydrotherapy:** Hydrotherapy's vast benefits range from stress reduction to improved circulation, making it a cornerstone of holistic healing. For beginners, the key is to start small and integrate simple practices into your routine. Begin with a comforting warm bath two nights a week, adding a few drops of lavender essential oil to enhance relaxation. This modest start not only introduces you to the benefits of hydrotherapy but also sets the foundation for a soothing bedtime ritual that promotes restful sleep.

- **Introducing Aromatherapy into Daily Routines:** Aromatherapy can significantly impact emotional and mental well-being with minimal effort, making it ideal for those new to holistic practices. Start by selecting one essential oil that resonates with you, such as citrus for energy or peppermint for focus. Use a diffuser in your living space or workplace for one hour each morning, creating an environment that supports your desired mood and cognitive state. This simple integration can serve as a daily reminder of your commitment to holistic health.

- **Exploring Reflexology with Focused Touch:** Reflexology provides a hands-on approach to stimulating the body's healing processes, perfect for beginners looking to incorporate touch into their healing plan. Identify one area of concern, such as headaches or digestive discomfort. Spend a few minutes each evening applying gentle pressure to the corresponding reflex points on your feet or hands, using a reflexology chart for guidance. This practice not only offers targeted relief but also fosters a deeper connection to your body.

- **Creating a Harmonious Balance:** The essence of a holistic healing plan lies in the harmonious integration of various therapies, tailored to individual needs and lifestyle. Draft a simple weekly schedule that incorporates hydrotherapy, aromatherapy, and reflexology into your routine, ensuring each practice aligns with specific health goals. For instance, dedicate Monday and Wednesday evenings to hydrotherapy, use aromatherapy during workdays, and practice reflexology before bed each night. Adjust the schedule based on your responses and preferences.

- **Monitoring and Adjusting Your Plan:** Embrace the journey of holistic healing with openness and curiosity, paying close attention to how your body and mind respond to these therapies. Keep a wellness journal to note observations, feelings, and any changes in your well-being. This reflective practice can illuminate patterns and guide necessary adjustments to your plan, ensuring it remains aligned with your evolving health needs.

- **Seeking Professional Guidance:** As you become more comfortable with these practices, consider consulting professionals in hydrotherapy, aromatherapy, and reflexology. Their expertise can offer personalized insights and enhance the effectiveness of your holistic healing plan. Schedule a consultation with a certified practitioner who can provide tailored advice and possibly introduce more advanced techniques, enriching your wellness journey.

By starting small, creating a balanced plan, and remaining attuned to your body's signals, you can seamlessly weave these practices into your daily routine, enhancing your path to holistic health. Remember, the journey to wellness is personal and evolving; allow yourself the flexibility to explore, adjust, and grow within your holistic healing plan.

Building a Personalized Healing Plan

Steps To Assess Your Holistic Health Status

Embarking on a journey toward holistic health requires a thoughtful assessment of one's current health status and a clear identification of areas for improvement. This foundational step ensures that the personalized healing plan you develop is tailored to meet your unique needs, fostering a path to wellness that is both effective and sustainable. This chapter guides you through the essential steps to assess your health comprehensively and pinpoint specific areas where changes can lead to significant health enhancements.

Step 1: Conduct a Holistic Health Inventory

Begin by taking a holistic inventory of your health, considering not just the physical aspect but also emotional, mental, and spiritual well-being. This can involve reflecting on various components of health, such as:

- **Physical Health:** Note any chronic conditions, pain points, energy levels, sleep quality, and overall physical fitness.

- **Emotional Well-being:** Assess your emotional state, including stress levels, mood patterns, and resilience in facing life's challenges.

- **Mental Health:** Consider cognitive functions like memory, concentration, and your general outlook on life.

- **Spiritual Wellness:** Reflect on your sense of purpose, connection to something greater than yourself, and how it influences your well-being.

Step 2: Identify Specific Health Goals

With a comprehensive understanding of your current health status, the next step is to identify specific areas for improvement. These goals can range from tangible objectives like losing weight or lowering blood pressure to more qualitative goals such as reducing stress or enhancing emotional resilience. Ensure these goals are SMART: Specific, Measurable, Achievable, Relevant, and Time-bound.

Step 3: Prioritize Your Goals

Given that resources and energy are finite, it's crucial to prioritize your health goals based on urgency and impact. For instance, addressing chronic pain or managing high stress levels might take precedence over other goals because of their significant impact on your overall quality of life. Prioritization helps focus your efforts and resources on areas that will provide the most substantial benefits.

Step 4: Research and Choose Appropriate Therapies

With your goals in mind, research therapies and practices that align with your needs. This might involve exploring conventional medical treatments, as well as complementary therapies like nutrition, exercise, hydrotherapy, aromatherapy, reflexology, or mindfulness practices. The key is to select therapies that resonate with your lifestyle, beliefs, and health objectives.

Step 5: Seek Professional Guidance

Consulting with healthcare professionals can provide valuable insights and help tailor your chosen therapies to fit your specific needs. This may involve working with a range of practitioners, from doctors and nutritionists to holistic therapists and fitness coaches, ensuring a well-rounded approach to your health plan.

Step 6: Develop a Detailed Action Plan

Translate your goals and chosen therapies into a detailed action plan. This plan should outline specific steps, timelines, and milestones, breaking down larger goals into manageable tasks. For example, if increasing physical activity is a goal, your plan might include scheduling three weekly workout sessions and tracking your progress.

Step 7: Implement, Monitor, and Adjust

With your personalized healing plan in place, the next step is implementation. Begin integrating the therapies and practices into your daily routine, staying mindful of your body's responses. Regular monitoring allows you to assess the effectiveness of your plan and make necessary adjustments. This iterative process ensures that your healing plan evolves with your health journey, remaining aligned with your changing needs and goals.

Creating a Personalized Healing Plan

Creating a personalized healing plan inspired by Barbara O'Neill's teachings involves embracing a holistic approach to health that prioritizes natural remedies, proper nutrition, and a balanced lifestyle. This checklist distills O'Neill's core teachings into practical ideas, enabling individuals to implement these principles into their own holistic healing plans effectively.

Adopt a Plant-Based Diet

- Gradually increase the intake of fruits, vegetables, whole grains, nuts, and seeds.

- Experiment with plant-based recipes that incorporate a wide variety of nutrient-dense foods.

- Plan meals that are colorful and diverse to ensure a broad spectrum of vitamins, minerals, and phytonutrients.

Incorporate Regular Physical Activity

- Integrate daily exercises that you enjoy, such as walking, yoga, swimming, or cycling.

- Explore the benefits of rebounding as a low-impact, high-efficiency exercise to stimulate lymphatic drainage and improve overall fitness.

- Set achievable fitness goals, such as a daily step count or specific yoga poses to master.

Utilize Natural Remedies for Common Ailments

- Create a home remedy kit with essential oils, herbal teas, and tinctures for addressing minor health issues like headaches, digestive discomfort, and stress.

- Learn to make simple herbal remedies, such as ginger tea for digestion or a lavender oil blend for relaxation.

Practice Detoxification Techniques

- Schedule regular detox periods, using methods such as juice fasting, herbal cleanses, or sauna sessions to support the body's natural detoxification processes.

- Include detox-supporting foods in your diet, like leafy greens, beets, and lemon water.

Enhance Well-being with Hydrotherapy

- Implement contrast showers or warm baths with Epsom salts to relieve muscle tension and promote relaxation.
- Use cold compresses for acute injuries to reduce inflammation and speed up recovery.

Prioritize Rest and Quality Sleep

- Establish a relaxing nighttime routine that may include reading, meditation, or aromatherapy to improve sleep quality.
- Maintain a consistent sleep schedule, aiming for 7-9 hours of restful sleep each night.

Implement Stress Reduction Techniques

- Practice daily mindfulness or meditation to manage stress levels and enhance emotional resilience.
- Find hobbies or activities that relax and rejuvenate your spirit, such as gardening, painting, or spending time in nature.

Monitor Your Progress and Adjust Accordingly

- Keep a health journal to track your diet, exercise, sleep patterns, and how you feel physically and emotionally.
- Regularly review your goals and the effectiveness of your healing plan, making adjustments as needed to continue supporting your health and well-being.

Seek Professional Guidance When Needed

- Consult with healthcare professionals, especially when integrating new supplements or making significant lifestyle changes.
- Consider working with a holistic health coach or naturopathic doctor to fine-tune your personalized healing plan.

By following this checklist, you can create a comprehensive and personalized healing plan that reflects Barbara O'Neill's holistic health teachings. This approach not only fosters physical health but also nurtures mental and emotional well-being, leading to a balanced and fulfilling lifestyle.

Adjusting The Plan As Circumstances Change

Adjusting your personalized healing plan as you progress and as circumstances change is crucial for maintaining its relevance and effectiveness over time. Adaptability ensures that your approach to wellness evolves in tandem with your body's needs, lifestyle shifts, and new health goals. This guidance provides practical strategies and examples, including suggested quantities where applicable, to help you fine-tune your holistic healing plan for maximum accuracy and reliability.

- **Assessing Progress Regularly:** Set a regular schedule for assessing your health and wellness progress. Every three to six months might be a realistic interval. Use a health journal to track changes in symptoms, energy levels, and overall well-being. For instance, note if your goal was to reduce stress levels and you've been practicing mindfulness for 15 minutes daily, assess changes in stress-related symptoms like sleep quality or anxiety episodes.

- **Listening to Your Body's Signals:** Become attuned to your body's feedback. If you've incorporated 30 minutes of rebounding into your routine five times a week and start feeling increased fatigue rather than vitality, consider adjusting the frequency to three times a week or reducing the session length to 20 minutes. This attentiveness allows you to respond to your body's needs dynamically.

- **Updating Goals Based on Life Changes:** Life events, such as a new job or a move, can significantly impact your daily routine and stress levels. If a job change leads to more sedentary hours, recalibrate your physical activity goals. For example, increase your daily step goal from 8,000 to 10,000 steps to counteract additional sitting time and incorporate stretching exercises every two hours to maintain flexibility and circulation.

- **Incorporating New Findings and Recommendations:** Stay informed about the latest research and recommendations in holistic health. If new studies suggest that consuming at least 25 grams of fiber daily can significantly benefit digestive health, review your dietary intake and adjust as needed to meet or exceed this recommendation. Incorporating a variety of fiber-rich foods, such as berries (8 grams of fiber per cup), lentils (15 grams per cup cooked), and chia seeds (10 grams per 2 tablespoons), can help you reach this target.

- **Adjusting Nutritional Needs:** As your body changes or as you age, your nutritional needs may shift. For instance, if you find your energy levels waning, you might need to reassess your iron intake, especially if following a plant-based diet. Adult men require about 8 mg of iron per day, while women until the age of 50 need about 18 mg. Consider adding more iron-rich plant foods, such as spinach (3.6 mg per 100g) or fortified cereals, and pair them with vitamin C-rich foods to enhance absorption.

- **Modifying Exercise Routines for Balance:** If your initial exercise routine focused heavily on cardio, but you're noticing a lack of strength gains, rebalance your routine to include strength training sessions at least twice a week. This adjustment ensures a comprehensive approach to physical fitness, addressing both cardiovascular health and muscle strength.

- **Tailoring Mindfulness Practices:** If you started with guided meditation to enhance mental well-being but find your focus waning, experiment with different forms of mindfulness practices. Transitioning to a silent meditation or trying mindfulness through movement, such as tai chi or mindful walking, can reignite your engagement with the practice. Starting with 10-minute sessions and gradually increasing to 20 minutes as you become more comfortable can help maintain consistency and interest.

Community and Support

+

In this healing journey, the importance of support cannot be overstated. It acts as a guiding light, providing warmth, encouragement, and a sense of shared humanity that can make all the difference. This chapter is a heartwarming exploration of the pivotal role that support plays in our healing journey, reminding us that we are not alone in our quest for wellness. In the tapestry of healing, each thread of support—be it from loved ones, healthcare professionals, or a community of like-minded individuals—adds strength and richness to the overall picture. It's a gentle reminder that healing is not a solitary endeavor but a shared journey that is enriched by the compassion, understanding, and care we receive and offer to others.

The Warm Embrace of Loved Ones: The support of family and friends offers a comforting embrace that can carry us through the toughest days. It's in the simple acts of kindness—a listening ear, a heartfelt conversation, or a shared meal—that we often find the strength to continue. These moments of connection not only lighten our burdens but also fill our healing journey with love and joy. Imagine the feeling of being understood and accepted in your most vulnerable moments; this is the gift of unconditional support from those we hold dear.

The Guiding Hand of Healthcare Professionals: Healthcare professionals who approach their work with compassion and empathy become invaluable allies in our journey. Their expertise, coupled with a genuine concern for our well-being, provides a beacon of hope and a trusted guide through the complexities of healing. They not only offer medical support but also validate our experiences and emotions, making the healing journey less daunting. The trust and rapport we build with our caregivers become cornerstones of our support system, empowering us to make informed decisions about our health with confidence.

The Collective Strength of Community: Finding a community of individuals who share similar health challenges or goals can be incredibly affirming. Whether it's a support group, an online forum, or a wellness class, these communal spaces offer a sense of belonging and understanding that is both healing and transformative. Sharing experiences, challenges, and victories with others fosters a collective resilience that uplifts and inspires. In these communities, we find not just support but also friendship, empathy, and a shared desire for growth and wellness.

Nurturing Self-Compassion: Amidst seeking support from others, it's essential to cultivate self-compassion. Being kind and gentle with ourselves, acknowledging our struggles without judgment, and honoring our needs and emotions are fundamental aspects of self-support. This inner compassion becomes a soothing balm, healing wounds and encouraging growth with the tender reminder that we are doing our best.

The journey toward healing is a mosaic of experiences, emotions, and encounters that shape our path to wellness. Support, in its many forms, is the golden thread that weaves through this mosaic, holding it together and giving it beauty and strength. It reminds us that healing is not just about the destination but also about the connections we make and the compassion we share along the way. In this journey, let us open our hearts to the support around us and within us, embracing the journey with hope, courage, and love.

Finding Communities Of Like-Minded People

Finding and engaging with communities of like-minded individuals offers a sense of belonging, understanding, and shared purpose that can significantly enhance our journey towards wellness. This chapter delves into the warmth and connection that these communities provide, guiding you on how to find and engage with groups that resonate with your healing path, and illustrating the profound impact they can have on your life.

Discovering Your Community

Identifying Your Interests and Needs: Begin by reflecting on your health goals, interests, and the type of support you seek. Whether it's a group focused on holistic health practices, a fitness community, or a support group for specific health conditions, understanding your needs is the first step in finding your tribe.

Research and Exploration: Utilize online platforms, social media, and health forums to research communities that align with your interests. Many wellness practitioners, yoga studios, and holistic health centers also offer workshops and groups that can serve as gateways to finding like-minded individuals.

Attend Events and Workshops: Participating in local workshops, seminars, and health-related events is a fantastic way to connect with potential communities. These gatherings not only provide valuable information but also the opportunity to meet people with similar interests in a natural, engaging setting.

Engaging with Your Community

Be Open and Authentic: When you find a community that feels right, approach it with openness and authenticity. Sharing your journey, listening to others, and participating actively creates a mutual exchange of support and understanding that strengthens the bonds within the community.

Volunteer and Contribute: Offering your time or skills to community activities can deepen your sense of belonging and investment. Whether it's assisting with event organization, sharing knowledge, or supporting new members, your contribution can enrich the community experience for everyone involved.

Create and Participate in Rituals: Many communities have rituals or regular meet-ups that strengthen their collective bond. Engage fully in these traditions, whether it's a weekly meditation circle, a monthly health potluck, or an annual wellness retreat. These rituals become cherished moments of connection and growth.

The Benefits of Community Engagement

Shared Knowledge and Experiences: Communities provide a rich tapestry of knowledge and personal stories that can offer insights, inspiration, and practical advice tailored to your healing journey.

Emotional Support and Encouragement: The emotional uplift that comes from being part of a supportive community is invaluable. Celebrating successes together, providing comfort during challenging times, and simply knowing you're not alone can make all the difference in your journey.

Accountability and Motivation: Engaging with a community can also foster a sense of accountability and motivation. The collective energy of a group focused on similar goals can propel you forward, keeping you motivated and on track with your wellness objectives.

Sustaining Engagement

Regular Participation: Consistency is key to building and maintaining connections within your community. Regular participation, whether in person or virtually, helps sustain the relationships and support network you've built.

- **Stay Connected:** In today's digital age, staying connected with your community can extend beyond physical meet-ups. Engage with community forums, social media groups, or newsletters to keep the sense of community alive, even when you're apart.

- **Reflect and Reassess:** As you grow and evolve on your healing journey, periodically reflect on your community engagement. Ensure that it continues to align with your needs and contributes positively to your journey. Don't hesitate to seek out new communities if your interests or goals shift.

Finding and engaging with a community of like-minded individuals offers a sanctuary of support, inspiration, and shared joy on the path to wellness. In these spaces, we not only find others who resonate with our journey but also discover deeper aspects of ourselves, fostering a connection that nourishes both the individual and the collective. As you navigate your path, remember that the strength of community lies not just in the support you receive but in the support you give, creating a beautiful cycle of healing, growth, and connection.

CONCLUSION

And just like that, we're wrapping up our adventure through Barbara O'Neill's world of holistic health, standing on the brink of something new and exciting in our quest to feel our best. Flipping through these pages, we didn't just learn a thing or two about getting back to basics with our health; we've actually started changing from the inside out. It's like we're at the start of a path that's going to require some patience, a lot of sticking to it, and a deep trust in the awesome power of healing from within and from the world around us. Barbara's been our guiding star, showing us how going natural can be simple but oh-so-effective. We've dived into the incredible ways our bodies can fix themselves, the healing hugs of Mother Nature, and finding that perfect balance for true well-being. These big ideas are now part of our toolkit on this healing journey—a journey that's as much about us as individuals as it is about all of us together.

As you step out on your own path to wellness, keep these lessons close. Be open to trying out all kinds of natural fixes, from the soothing power of water therapy to the gentle guidance of aromatherapy and reflexology. Every method, every bit of advice, is a chance to change your life in big and small ways. But remember, this path to natural healing is more than just collecting tips; it's about giving it time, keeping at it, and staying open to where it leads you. Sure, there'll be tough spots and times you wonder if you're on the right track. When that happens, lean on your inner strength, the support network around you, and the always-available healing touch of nature.

Let this be a journey of finding out more about yourself, how resilient you are, how much you can grow, and just how powerful your own healing abilities are. What you've learned isn't just a way to better health; it's an invite to connect more deeply with life, to live more fully and vibrantly. On the holistic health road, every little choice, every step in sync with nature's rhythm, is a healing act. This healing journey is one we're all on together, each step a yes to life's amazing capacity to renew and change. As you move forward, let Barbara O'Neill's wisdom encourage you to keep exploring, learning, and expanding. Let it show you that the real magic isn't just about reaching a certain destination or achieving perfect health, but in the journey itself and the love and understanding we grow for ourselves and the world along the way.

The true magic of natural health methods and holistic practices is in how they transform not just our bodies but our hearts and minds, leading us to a life filled with wellness, balance, and joy. So, with these insights lighting your way, step boldly into your own natural healing journey. Approach each day with wonder and thankfulness, knowing every step is taking you closer to the radiant health and wholeness you're meant for. This path is yours to travel, and its treasures are yours to find.

Welcome to your transformative journey.

Made in the USA
Las Vegas, NV
10 June 2024

90949654R00052